Pediatric Code
Crosswalk
ICD-9-CM to *ICD-10-CM*

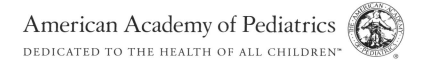

Transitioning to **10**

Editor

Jeffrey F. Linzer, Sr, MD, FAAP

AAP Representative, *ICD-9-CM* Editorial Advisory Board
Member, Committee on Coding and Nomenclature
American Academy of Pediatrics

American Academy of Pediatrics
DEDICATED TO THE HEALTH OF ALL CHILDREN™

For additional copies or information about other AAP coding resources, contact

American Academy of Pediatrics
141 Northwest Point Blvd
Elk Grove Village, IL 60007-1019

Library of Congress Control Number: 2012947275
ISBN: 978-1-58110-737-1

MA0629
11-94

Pediatric Code Crosswalk: ICD-9-CM to ICD-10-CM is designed as a quick reference for pediatric diagnosis coding. At the time of release, only *International Classification of Diseases, Ninth Revision, Clinical Modification (ICD-9-CM)* codes are valid for use; therefore, everything is still listed first under its *ICD-9-CM* code and terminology. First, review the Basic Coding Guidelines for *ICD-9-CM* (page v). Next, determine the *ICD-9-CM* classification that would most likely include the diagnosis to be coded and turn to that class in the crosswalk.

Search for the diagnosis in the class alphabetic listing by using the key word in the diagnosis. If not found, search by all other words that might relate to the diagnosis. Some diagnoses may not be found in the class where you might expect and may be found immediately following the class under "Other Related Diagnoses."

Diagnoses printed in *italic* on the *ICD-9-CM* side are nonspecific and somewhat generic. More detailed codes have been left out for space considerations. These codes may be helpful in coding for minor or unlisted complaints, findings, or diagnoses. Refer to the *ICD-9-CM* book for more detailed information concerning these codes.

While *ICD-9-CM* coding guidelines designate several V codes as primary diagnoses, payment rules vary with third-party payers. Check with your local payer as to which codes are recognized under the guidelines.

For this edition, *International Classification of Diseases, 10th Revision, Clinical Modification (ICD-10-CM)* codes have been included. Note that these codes are not to be reported until after the approved implementation date. At time of publication this date was set for October 1, 2014. These codes are to be used for reference, training, and education purposes only. It is vital that your practice begin to learn the *ICD-10-CM* code set and how it will differ from *ICD-9-CM*. *ICD-9-CM* codes were crosswalked into the *ICD-10-CM* code set using General Equivalence Mappings developed by the Centers for Disease Control and Prevention. Other resources were also used in crosswalking the 2 code sets; therefore, this crosswalk should be looked at as the American Academy of Pediatrics interpretation.

Jeffrey F. Linzer, Sr, MD, FAAP

Editor
AAP Representative, *ICD-9-CM* Editorial Advisory Board
Member, Committee on Coding and Nomenclature
American Academy of Pediatrics

ICD-9-CM Classification

Basic Coding Guidelines for *ICD-9-CM*

1. Select appropriate *International Classification of Diseases, Ninth Revision, Clinical Modification (ICD-9-CM)* code(s) **001.0** through **V89.09** to identify diagnosis, symptoms, conditions, problems, complaints, or other reasons for the patient encounter.

2. Code to the highest degree of specificity. Assign the fourth or fifth digit when indicated.

3. Diagnoses documented as *probable, suspected, questionable,* or *rule out* should not be coded as if the diagnosis is confirmed (in the outpatient setting). Code to the highest degree of certainty for the encounter, such as symptoms, signs, abnormal test results, or other reasons for the visit.

4. List the *ICD-9-CM* code that is identified as the main reason for the procedure or service first in the medical record. Next, list any current coexisting conditions, if those conditions affect the treatment or management of the patient.

5. A chronic disease treated on an ongoing basis may be coded and reported as many times as it is applicable to the patient's treatment.

6. Do not code conditions that were previously treated and no longer exist at the time of the encounter.

7. When only ancillary diagnostic or therapeutic services are provided, list the diagnosis or problem for which the services are being provided and next list the appropriate V code for the services.

8. E codes are never used alone or as principal diagnosis codes. E codes may be assigned to any *ICD-9-CM* code **001.0–999.9.**

9. For surgical procedures, use the applicable diagnosis code. If the postoperative diagnosis is different from the preoperative diagnosis, use the *ICD-9-CM* code for the postoperative diagnosis.

Introduction

Pediatric Code Crosswalk: ICD-9-CM to ICD-10-CM was designed as a guide for pediatricians to be used in association with volumes 1 and 2 of the *2013 International Classification of Diseases, Ninth Revision, Clinical Modification (ICD-9-CM)*. *ICD-9-CM,* which has been in use in the United States since 1977, is revised annually. Currently there is a freeze on the introduction of new *ICD-9-CM* and *International Classification of Diseases, 10th Revision, Clinical Modification (ICD-10-CM)* codes unless the *ICD* Coordination and Maintenance Committee determines they meet the criteria for a new disease. For 2012 there were no new *ICD-9-CM* codes added for pediatrics.

   The diagnoses and diseases listed in this coding crosswalk have been identified as some of the most commonly encountered in pediatric patients, and the corresponding *ICD-9-CM* codes reflect these diagnoses and diseases. However, the *ICD-9-CM* codes in this crosswalk also may be used to report other diagnoses and diseases not listed here.

   The American Academy of Pediatrics (AAP) will continue to monitor changes to the *ICD-9-CM* and *ICD-10-CM* code sets carefully and distribute the information in a timely manner to the membership through various means, including the annual publication of this guide with significant revisions related to primary care pediatrics.

Disclaimer
Pediatric Code Crosswalk: ICD-9-CM to ICD-10-CM has been designed to be a guide to be used with *ICD-9-CM*. While every effort has been made to ensure the accuracy of the information in this crosswalk, the AAP does not guarantee that this guide is accurate, complete, or without error. The recommendations in this publication do not indicate an exclusive course of treatment or serve as a standard of medical care. Variations, taking into account individual circumstances, may be appropriate. It is important to note that *ICD-10-CM* codes are not currently valid and should not be reported until implemented by the Centers for Medicare & Medicaid Services.

Acknowledgment
Appreciation is extended to the members and staff of the Committee on Coding and Nomenclature for their input and critiques of the crosswalk, most notably Becky Dolan, MPH, CPC, CPEDC, and Teri Salus, MPA, CPC, CPEDC.

ICD-9-CM Symbols

*   Code underlying condition/ cause/disease first

\+   Use additional code(s) to identify manifestations

§   Use E code to identify agent or cause

ICD-10-CM Symbols

*   Use another code first to identify underlying condition/ cause/disease

\+   Code listed here is to be used first along with additional codes to identify, eg, manifestations

\-   Refer to *ICD-10-CM* manual for specific code

√   Report with seventh digit code to define encounter

±   Additional digit required

▲   Last digit – 0 = Unspec
                  1 = Right
                  2 = Left
                  3 = Bilateral

¤   Last digit – 1 = Right
                  2 = Left
                  3 = Bilateral
                  9 = Unspec

∞   Code as listed is Unspec Report with last digit of 1 = Right or 2 = Left if known

£   Combination code in *ICD-10-CM*

Key to Abbreviations

ADD	Attention-Deficit Disorder
AIDS	Acquired Immunodeficiency Syndrome
ALPS	Autoimmune Lymphoproliferative Syndrome
ALTE	Apparent Life-Threatening Event
ARDS	Adult Respiratory Distress Syndrome
ASA	Acetylsalicylic Acid
ATV	All-Terrain Vehicle
BMI	Body Mass Index
BP	Blood Pressure
CNS	Central Nervous System
CSF	Cerebrospinal Fluid
DIC	Disseminated Intravascular Coagulation
DT	Diphtheria and Tetanus
DTaP	Diphtheria, Tetanus, and Acellular Pertussis
DTP	Diphtheria, Tetanus, and Pertussis
Exam	Examination
FNHTR	Febrile Nonhemolytic Transfusion Reaction
Fx	Fracture
g	Grams
G6PD	Glucose-6-Phosphate Dehydrogenase
GI	Gastrointestinal
GU	Genitourinary
Hb	Hemoglobin
Hib	Haemophilus influenzae type b (Vaccine)
HIV	Human Immunodeficiency Virus
HPV	Human Papillomavirus
Hx	History
IUD	Intrauterine Device
LBW	Low Birth Weight
LOC	Loss of Consciousness
MCLS	Mucocutaneous Lymph Node Syndrome
MMR	Measles, Mumps, and Rubella

MRSA	Methicillin-resistant Staphylococcus aureus
MSSA	Methicillin-susceptible Staphylococcus aureus
N/A	A Code Does Not Exist for This Diagnosis in This Code Set
NEC	Not Elsewhere Classified
NOS	No Other Symptoms
Obs	Observation
PICC	Peripherally Inserted Central Catheter
PTSD	Post-traumatic Stress Disorder
RSV	Respiratory Syncytial Virus
SIADH	Syndrome of Inappropriate Antidiuretic Hormone
SQ	Subcutaneous
STD	Sexually Transmitted Disease
STEC	Shiga Toxin–Producing E coli
Strep	Streptococcal
Sx	Symptoms
TACO	Transfusion-Associated Circulatory Overload
TAR	Thrombocytopenia–Absent Radius
TB	Tuberculosis
Td	Tetanus and Diphtheria Toxoids
Tdap	Tetanus, Diphtheria, and Acellular Pertussis
TMJ	Temporomandibular Joint
TRALI	Transfusion Related to Acute Lung Injury
Unspec	Unspecified
URI	Upper Respiratory Infection
UTI	Urinary Tract Infection
VA	Ventriculoatrial
VP	Ventriculoperitoneal
vs	Versus
w/	With
w/o	Without
X	Additional Fourth or Fifth Digit Required (ONLY When Following *ICD-9-CM* Code)

Transitioning to 10

1. Infectious and Parasitic Diseases

ICD-10-CM codes are not valid for use at the time of publication and should not be reported until the official implementation date set by the Centers for Medicare & Medicaid Services.

ICD-9-CM		ICD-10-CM	
006.0	Amebiasis, Acute	A06.0	
038.3	Anaerobic Septicemia	A41.4	
022.0	Anthrax, Cutaneous	A22.0	
022.2	Anthrax, GI	A22.2	
022.1	Anthrax, Pulmonary	A22.1	
127.0	Ascariasis, Unspec	B77.9	
005.1	Botulism, Food Poisoning	A05.1	
040.41	Botulism, Infant	A48.51	
040.42	Botulism, Wound	A48.52+	*for wound*
008.43	Campylobacter Enteritis	A04.5	
112.0	Candida, Oral (Thrush)	B37.0	excludes neonatal
		P37.5	neonatal
112.84	Candidal Esophagitis	B37.81	
112.1	Candidal Vulvovaginitis	B37.3	
112.3	Candidiasis of Skin and Nails	B37.2	
112.5	Candidiasis, Systemic+	B37.7	
078.3	Cat-scratch Disease	A28.1	
052.9	Chickenpox w/o Complications	B01.9	
133.8	Chiggers	B88.0	
077.98	Chlamydia Conjunctivitis	A74.89	excludes neonatal
		P39.1	neonatal
099.55	Chlamydia, GU, Unspec	A56.2	
079.98	Chlamydia, Unspec (Non-STD)	A74.9	

1. Infectious and Parasitic Diseases *(cont)*

ICD-9-CM		ICD-10-CM
099.41	Chlamydia Urethritis (STD)	A56.01
077.99	Conjunctivitis, Viral, Unspec	B30.9
078.5	Cytomegaloviral Disease, Unspec	B25.9
110.9	Dermatophytosis, Ringworm	B39.5
009.2	Diarrhea/Dysentery, Infectious	A09
009.3	Diarrhea, Presumed Infectious	A09
008.00	E. coli Enteritis, Unspec	A04.4
008.04	E. coli, Enterohemorrhagic	A04.3
008.01	E. coli, Enteropathogenic	A04.0
008.02	E. coli, Enterotoxigenic	A04.1
082.40	Ehrlichiosis	A77.40
062.5	Encephalitis, California	A83.5
062.2	Encephalitis, Eastern	A83.2
054.3	Encephalitis, Herpes	B10.09
052.0	Encephalitis, Post-chickenpox	B01.11
062.3	Encephalitis, St Louis	A83.3
049.9	*Encephalitis, Viral*	A86
066.41	Encephalitis, West Nile	A92.31
N/A	Enterovirus, Enteritis	A08.39
035	Erysipelas	A46
058.10	Exanthema Subitum (Sixth Disease)	B08.20
057.0	Fifth Disease	B08.3
005.9	Food Poisoning, Unspec	A05.9
N/A	Gastroenteritis, Acute, Viral	A08.4
009.0	Gastroenteritis, Infectious	A09
009.1	Gastroenteritis, Presumed Infectious	N/A
054.10	Genital Herpes, Unspec	A60.00
007.1	Giardiasis	A07.1
098.15	Gonococcal Cervicitis	A54.03
098.40	Gonococcal Newborn Conjunctivitis	A54.31
098.17	Gonococcal Salpingitis	A54.24

ICD-9-CM		ICD-10-CM	
Ø98.Ø	Gonorrhea, Acute	A54.ØØ	
	Gonococcal Urethritis	A54.Ø1	
	Gonococcal Vulvovaginitis	A54.Ø2	
Ø38.4Ø	Gram-negative Septicemia	A41.5Ø	Gram-negative Sepsis
Ø38.41	H. influenzae Sepsis	A41.3*	Sepsis Due to H. influenzae
Ø74.3	Hand, Foot, and Mouth Disease	BØ8.4	
Ø7Ø.1	Hepatitis A, w/o Hepatic Coma	B15.9	
Ø7Ø.3Ø	Hepatitis B, Acute w/o Hepatic Coma	B16.9	
Ø7Ø.51	Hepatitis C, Acute w/o Hepatic Coma	B17.1Ø	
Ø7Ø.54	Hepatitis C, Chronic w/o Hepatic Coma	B18.2	Viral Hepatitis C, Chronic
Ø7Ø.9	Hepatitis, Unspec, w/o Hepatic Coma	B17.9	Acute, Unspec, w/o Hepatic Coma
		B19.9	Unspec, w/o Hepatic Coma
Ø74.Ø	Herpangina	BØ8.5	
Ø54.1Ø	Herpes, Genital, Unspec	A6Ø.ØØ	
Ø54.9	Herpes Simplex, NOS	BØØ.9	
Ø53.9	Herpes Zoster/Shingles	BØ2.9	
Ø54.2	Herpetic Gingivostomatitis	BØØ.2	
Ø54.6	Herpetic Whitlow	BØØ.89	
Ø42	HIV Disease (AIDS), Symptomatic+	B2Ø*	
Ø75	Infectious Mononucleosis	B27.9Ø	Unspec w/o Complications
Ø27.Ø	Listeriosis	A32.Ø-	
Ø88.81	Lyme Disease	A69.2-	
Ø84.6	Malaria	B54	
Ø55.9	Measles	BØ5.9	
Ø47.Ø	Meningitis, Coxsackie	A87.Ø	Meningitis, Enteroviral, Coxsackie
Ø47.8	Meningitis Due to Specific Virus	A87.8	Meningitis, Viral, Other
	Enterovirus	A87.Ø	
Ø54.72	Meningitis, Herpes Simplex	BØØ.3	
Ø47.9	*Meningitis, Viral/Aseptic*	A87.9	Meningitis, Viral, Unspec
		GØ3.Ø	Meningitis, Aseptic

1. Infectious and Parasitic Diseases *(cont)*

ICD-9-CM		ICD-10-CM	
Ø36.9	Meningococcal Infection	A39.9	
Ø36.Ø	Meningococcal Meningitis	A39.Ø	
Ø36.2	Meningococcemia	A39.4	
Ø78.Ø	Molluscum Contagiosum	BØ8.1	
Ø38.12	MRSA Septicemia	A41.Ø*	
Ø38.11	MSSA Septicemia	A41.Ø*	
Ø72.9	Mumps	B26.9	
Ø52.2	Myelitis, Post-chickenpox	BØ1.12	
Ø57.8	Parascarlatina/Scarlatiniform	BØ9	Viral Exanthem, Unspec
		L44.4	Infantile Papular Acrodermatosis
129	Parasitism, Intestinal, Unspec	B82.9	
Ø79.83	Parvovirus B19	B34.3	
132.1	Pediculosis, Body	B85.1	
132.2	Pediculosis, Genital	B85.3	
132.Ø	Pediculosis, Head	B85.Ø	
Ø33.9	Pertussis/Whooping Cough	A37.9Ø	Whooping Cough, Unspec, w/o Pneumonia
		A37.91	w/ Pneumonia
127.4	Pinworm	B8Ø	
Ø38.2	Pneumococcal Septicemia	A4Ø.3	
Ø71	Rabies	A82.9	Rabies, Unspec
Ø82.Ø	Rocky Mountain Spotted Fever	A77.Ø	
Ø58.1Ø	Roseola Infantum	BØ8.2Ø	
ØØ8.61	Rotavirus Enteritis	AØ8.Ø	
Ø56.9	Rubella	BØ6.9	
ØØ3.Ø	Salmonella Gastroenteritis	AØ2.2	
ØØ3.8	Salmonellosis	AØ2.8	
135	Sarcoidosis	D86.-	
133.Ø	Scabies	B86	
Ø34.1	Scarlet Fever/Scarlatina	A38.9	Uncomplicated, NOS
		A38.Ø	w/ Otitis Media
		A38.8	w/ Other Complications
Ø38.9	Septicemia, Unspec	A41.9	Septicemia, NOS
ØØ4.9	Shigellosis	AØ3.9	

ICD-9-CM		ICD-10-CM	
099.9	*STD, Unspec*	A64	
038.0	Strep Septicemia	A40.9	Strep Septicemia, Unspec
034.0	Strep Sore Throat	J02.0	Strep Pharyngitis/Sore Throat
		J03.00	Strep Tonsillitis, Acute
		J03.01	Strep Tonsillitis, Recurrent
120.3	Swimmer's Itch	B65.3	
090.2	Syphilis, Congenital	A50.2	
091.0	Syphilis, Genital (Primary)	A51.0	
097.1	Syphilis, Latent	A53.0	
091.2	Syphilis, Other Primary	A51.2	
123.9	*Tapeworm*	B71.9	
017.20	TB Adenitis	A18.2	TB Peripheral Lymphadenopathy
013.00	TB Meningitis	A17.0	
011.90	TB, Pulmonary	A15.9	TB, Pulmonary, Unspec
110.0	Tinea capitis (Scalp)	B35.0	
110.5	Tinea corporis (Body)	B35.4	
110.3	Tinea cruris (Groin)	B35.6	
110.4	Tinea pedis (Feet)	B35.3	
111.0	Tinea versicolor	B36.0	
040.82	Toxic Shock Syndrome	A48.3	
130.9	Toxoplasmosis	B58.9	
131.09	Trichomonal Cervicitis	A59.09	
131.02	Trichomonal Urethritis	A59.03	
131.01	Trichomonal Vulvovaginitis	A59.01	
099.40	Urethritis, Nonspecific (STD)	N34.1	
057.9	Viral Exanthem	B09	Viral Exanthem, NOS
079.99	Viral Infection, Unspec	B97.89	
078.19	Warts, Common	B07.8	
078.11	Warts, Genital	A63.0	
078.12	Warts, Plantar	B07.0	
066.40	West Nile Fever, w/o Complications	A92.30	

1. Infectious and Parasitic Diseases *(cont)*

ICD-9-CM		ICD-10-CM	
For Use With Bacterial Infection With Specified Conditions			
Ø41.84	Anaerobes	B97.Ø	
Ø41.42	E. coli Non-O157 STEC	B96.2	
Ø41.49	E. coli, Non-STEC	B96.2	
Ø41.41	E. coli O157 STEC	B96.2	
Ø41.43	E. coli STEC, Unspec	B96.2	
Ø41.85	Gram-negative aerobes	N/A	
Ø41.5	H. influenzae	B96.3	
Ø41.86	Helicobacter pylori	B96.81	
Ø41.12	MRSA	B95.6	
Ø41.11	MSSA	B95.6	
Ø41.81	Mycoplasma	B96.Ø	
Ø41.2	Pneumococcus	B95.3*	*specific disease classified elsewhere*
Ø41.6	Proteus	B96.4	
Ø41.7	Pseudomonas	B96.5	
Ø41.Ø4	Streptococcus, Enterococcus	B95.2	
Ø41.Ø1	Streptococcus, Group A	B95.Ø	
Ø41.Ø2	Streptococcus, Group B	B95.1	
Ø41.ØØ	Streptococcus, Unspec	B95.5	

ICD-9-CM		ICD-10-CM	
For Use to Identify Viral/Chlamydial Infection With Specified Conditions			
Ø79.Ø	Adenovirus	B97.Ø	
Ø79.88	Chlamydia, Other Specified	N/A	
Ø79.2	Coxsackievirus	B97.11	
Ø79.1	Echovirus	B97.12	
Ø79.3	Rhinovirus	N/A	
Ø79.89	Virus, Other Specified Enterovirus	B97.89	Enterovirus, Other Specified
		B97.1Ø	Enterovirus, Unspec

ICD-9-CM		ICD-10-CM	
Other Related Diagnoses			
795.31	Anthrax, Nonspecific Positive Findings	R89.9	Abnormal Finding, Unspec, Anthrax
488.Ø1	Avian Flu	JØ9.Ø1Ø	
771.83	Bacteremia, Newborn	R78.81	Bacteremia
466.11	Bronchiolitis, RSV	J21.Ø	

ICD-9-CM		ICD-10-CM	
771.7	Candidal Infection of Newborn Monilia Thrush	P37.5	
VØ2.7	Carrier, Gonorrhea	Z22.4	
VØ2.61	Carrier, Hepatitis B	Z22.51	
VØ2.62	Carrier, Hepatitis C	Z22.52	
VØ2.6Ø	Carrier, Hepatitis Unspec	Z22.5Ø	
VØ2.59	Carrier, Meningococcus or Other Specified Bacterial Disease	Z22.31	Carrier, Meningococcus
		Z22.8	Carrier, Other Specified
VØ2.54	Carrier, MRSA	Z22.32	
VØ2.53	Carrier, MSSA	Z22.32	
VØ2.8	Carrier, Other STD	Z22.4	
VØ2.52	Carrier, Streptococcus, Not Group B	Z22.338	
78Ø.64	Chills w/o Fever	R68.83	
372.ØØ	Conjunctivitis, Acute	H1Ø.3▲	
771.6	Conjunctivitis/Dacryocystitis, Newborn	P39.1	
372.Ø3	Conjunctivitis, Purulent	H1Ø.Ø2¤	
787.91	Diarrhea (Noninfectious)	R19.7	
VØ9.1	Drug-resistant Infection, Cephalosporins/ß-Lactams	Z16*	
VØ9.81	Drug-resistant Infection, Multiple Agents	Z16*	
VØ9.Ø	Drug-resistant Infection, Penicillin, MRSA	Z16*	
VØ9.9Ø	*Drug-resistant Infection, Single Agent*	Z16*	
VØ9.8Ø	Drug-resistant Infection, Vancomycin	Z16*	
323.61	Encephalitis, Infectious Acute Disseminated*	GØ4.ØØ	
323.62	Encephalitis, Other Postinfectious*	GØ4.3Ø	

1. Infectious and Parasitic Diseases *(cont)*

ICD-9-CM		ICD-10-CM	
Other Related Diagnoses *(cont)*			
VØ1.81	Exposure to Anthrax	**Z2Ø.81Ø**	
VØ1.83	Exposure to E. coli	**Z2Ø.Ø1**	
VØ1.84	Exposure to Meningococcus	**Z2Ø.811**	
VØ1.89	*Exposure to Other Communicable Disease*	**Z2Ø.89**	
VØ1.79	*Exposure to Other Viral Disease*	**Z2Ø.828**	
	Exposure to Hepatitis	**Z2Ø.5**	
	Exposure to HIV	**Z2Ø.6**	
VØ1.5	Exposure to Rabies	**Z2Ø.3**	
VØ1.4	Exposure to Rubella	**Z2Ø.4**	
VØ1.6	Exposure to STD	**Z2Ø.2**	
VØ1.1	Exposure to TB	**Z2Ø.1**	
VØ1.71	Exposure to Varicella	**Z2Ø.82Ø**	
778.4	Fever, Newborn	**P81.9**	Fever, Newborn, NOS
78Ø.61	Fever Presenting w/ (Chronic) Conditions Classified Elsewhere*	**R5Ø.81***	
78Ø.6Ø	Fever (w/ or w/o Chills)	**R5Ø.9**	
558.9	Gastroenteritis, Acute, Noninfectious	**K52.89**	Other Specified
		K52.9	Unspec
571.49	Hepatitis, Chronic Nonviral	**K73.2**	Hepatitis, Chronic Lobular, NEC
774.4	Hepatitis, Neonatal	**P59.29**	Hepatitis, Neonatal (Jaundice), Due to Other Hepatocellular Damage (Giant Cell Hepatitis)
		P59.2Ø	Hepatitis, Neonatal (Jaundice), Due to Unspec Hepatocellular Damage
		P59.1	Inspissated Bile Syndrome
VØ8	HIV Infection w/o Sx	**Z21**	
795.71	HIV Test, Nonspecific Results	**R75**	HIV Test, Inconclusive
78Ø.65	Hypothermia Not Associated w/ Low Environmental Temperature	**R68.Ø**	
999.9	*Immunization Complication/ Reaction* add E879.8 as secondary code	**T8Ø.62X√**	

ICD-9-CM		ICD-10-CM	
771.2	Infection, Congenital, Other (Specific)	P37.8	
	Herpes	P35.2	
	Toxoplasmosis	P37.1	
	Listeriosis	P37.2	
771.89	Infection, Other, During Perinatal Period	P39.8	
488.82	Influenza, Novel A	J10.1	
488.89	Influenza, Novel A w/ Other Manifestations	J10.89	
446.1	Kawasaki Disease/MCLS	M30.3	
320.9	Meningitis, Bacterial Unspec	G00.9	
320.82	Meningitis, Gram-negative	G00.9	
320.0	Meningitis, H. influenzae	G00.0	
320.1	Meningitis, Pneumococcal	G00.1	
320.2	Meningitis, Strep	G00.2	
V12.04	MRSA Infection, Hx of	Z86.14	
323.63	Myelitis, Postinfectious*	G04.89	
V71.82	Obs for Suspected Anthrax Exposure	Z03.810	
V71.83	Obs for Suspected Biologic Agent Exposure	Z03.818	
V71.89	Obs for Suspected Condition Evaluation for Meningitis Evaluation for Septicemia	Z03.89	
V29.0	Obs for Suspected Infection, Newborn Evaluation for Sepsis/Infection	P00.2	
V71.2	Obs for Suspected TB	Z03.89	
420.99	Pericarditis, Acute Purulent	I30.8	Pericarditis, Acute, Other
420.91	Pericarditis, Acute Viral	I30.0	
780.63	Postvaccination Fever	R50.83	
390	Rheumatic Fever	I00	
391.9	*Rheumatic Heart Disease*	I01.9	Rheumatic Heart Disease, Unspec
771.0	Rubella, Congenital	P35.0	

1. Infectious and Parasitic Diseases *(cont)*

ICD-9-CM		ICD-10-CM	
Other Related Diagnoses *(cont)*			
995.91	Sepsis	**A41.9**	
771.81	Sepsis, Newborn	**P36.0-**	
995.92	Sepsis, Severe	**R65.20***	Sepsis, Severe, w/o Septic Shock
785.52	Shock, Septic add 995.92 if organ dysfunction present	**R65.21***	Sepsis, Severe, w/ Septic Shock
998.02	Shock, Septic Postoperative* add 995.92 if organ dysfunction present	**T81.12X√**	
795.52	TB Cellular Immunity Test, Nonspecific Reaction w/o Active TB	**R76.12**	
V12.01	TB, Hx of	**Z86.11**	
795.51	TB Skin Test Positive w/o Active TB	**R76.11**	
597.80	Urethritis, Non-STD	**N34.1**	
771.82	UTI, Newborn	**P39.3**	
997.31	Ventilator-Associated Pneumonia	**J95.851+**	*to identify organism*

2. Neoplasms

ICD-10-CM codes are not valid for use at the time of publication and should not be reported until the official implementation date set by the Centers for Medicare & Medicaid Services.

ICD-9-CM		ICD-10-CM	
239.2	Bone Tumor, Unspec	D49.2	
170.7	Ewing Sarcoma, Lower Limb	C40.2-	
170.4	Ewing Sarcoma, Upper Limb	C40.0-	
212.7	Heart Tumor, Benign	D15.1	
228.01	Hemangioma, Skin	D18.01	
228.00	*Hemangioma, Unspec Site Cavernous Hemangioma*	D18.00	
204.00	Leukemia, Acute Lymphoblast	C91.00	
204.02	Leukemia, Acute Lymphoblast, Relapse	C91.02	
204.01	Leukemia, Acute Lymphoblast, Remission	C91.01	
205.00	Leukemia, Acute Myeloid	C92.00	
205.02	Leukemia, Acute Myeloid, Relapse	C92.02	
205.01	Leukemia, Acute Myeloid, Remission	C92.01	
214.1	Lipoma, Non-face, Skin/SQ	D17.30	
201.90	Lymphoma, Hodgkin	C81.90	
200.70	Lymphoma, Large Cell	C83.39	
202.80	Lymphoma, Non-Hodgkin	C85.9-	
202.70	Lymphoma, Peripheral T-cell	C84.40	
191.6	Medulloblastoma	C71.6	
191.5	Neoplasm Brain Ventricle	C71.5	
194.0	Neuroblastoma	C74.90∞	
237.71	Neurofibromatosis Type 1 von Recklinghausen Disease	Q85.01	
237.72	Neurofibromatosis Type 2 (Acoustic)	Q85.02	
237.70	Neurofibromatosis, Unspec	Q85.00	
216.9	Nevus, Unspec Site Pigmented, Skin, Giant, Hairy, Mole(s)	D23.9	
199.2	Organ Transplant-Associated Malignancy	C80.2*	*complication of transplant T86.-*
211.3	Polyposis, Familial	D12.6	

2. Neoplasms *(cont)*

ICD-9-CM		ICD-10-CM	
238.77	Post-transplant Lymphoproliferative Disorder	D47.Z1*	complication of transplanted organs and tissues T86.-
237.73	Schwannomatosis	Q85.03	
239.9	Tumor, Neoplastic Unspec	D49.9	
189.0	Wilms Tumor	C64.2	Left Kidney
		C64.1	Right Kidney
		C64.9	Unspec Kidney

Other Related Diagnoses			
789.30	*Abdominal/Umbilical Mass/ Swelling*	R19.00	
V10.81	Bone Tumor, Hx of	Z85.830	
V10.85	Brain Tumor, Hx of	Z85.841	
611.72	Breast Lump or Mass	N63	
V10.61	Leukemia, Lymphoid, Hx of	Z85.6	
V10.63	Leukemia, Monocytic, Hx of	Z85.6	
V10.62	Leukemia, Myeloid, Hx of	Z85.6	
V10.72	Lymphoma, Hodgkin, Hx of	Z85.71	
V10.71	Lymphoma, Non-Hodgkin, Hx of	Z85.72	
V10.88	Neuroblastoma, Hx of	Z85.858	
731.0	Paget Disease	M88.-	
569.0	Polyp, Rectal	K62.1	
V10.84	Retinoblastoma, Hx of	Z85.840	
V76.11	Screening Mammography, High-risk	Z12.31	
608.89	Scrotal/Testicular Mass	N44.2	Scrotal/Testicular Cyst
782.2	*Skin Mass/Lump/Nodule*	R22.-	by site
625.8	Vulvar Mass	N94.89	
V10.52	Wilms Tumor, Hx of	Z85.528	

3. Endocrine, Nutritional and Metabolic Diseases, and Immunity Disorders

ICD-10-CM codes are not valid for use at the time of publication and should not be reported until the official implementation date set by the Centers for Medicare & Medicaid Services.

ICD-9-CM		ICD-10-CM	
253.Ø	Acromegaly/Gigantism Sotos Syndrome	E22.Ø	
255.41	Addison Disease/Glucocorticoid Deficiency	E27.1	Addison Disease
		E27.49	Glucocorticoid Deficiency
	Adrenal Crisis	E27.2	Adrenal Crisis
255.2	Adrenogenital Syndrome	E25.9	
	Congenital Adrenal Hyperplasia	E25.Ø	
279.41	ALPS	D89.82	
27Ø.8	Amino-Acid Metabolic Disorder	E72.8	
	Lowe Syndrome	E72.Ø3+	*associated glaucoma H42.-*
259.52	Androgen Insensitivity, Partial	E34.52	
259.51	Androgen Insensitivity Syndrome	E34.51	
279.49	Autoimmune Disease, Unspec	D89.89	
277.4	Bilirubin Excretion Disorders	E8Ø.7	
	Crigler-Najjar Syndrome	E8Ø.5	
	Dubin-Johnson Syndrome	E8Ø.6	
269.3	Calcium Dietary Deficiency	E58	
277.82	Carnitine Deficiency Due to Inborn Errors of Metabolism	E71.42+	*associated inborn errors of metabolism*
277.83	Carnitine Deficiency, Iatrogenic	E71.43	
277.84	Carnitine Deficiency, Other (Secondary)	E71.448	
277.81	Carnitine Deficiency, Primary	E71.41	
279.2	Combined Immunodeficiency	D81.9	refer to *ICD-10-CM* for more specific code
255.Ø	Cushing Syndrome	E24.Ø	Primary (Pituitary)
		E24.2+	Secondary (Drug Induced) *to identify drug T36–T5Ø*
277.Ø3	Cystic Fibrosis w/ GI Sx	E84.19	
277.Ø1	Cystic Fibrosis w/ Meconium Ileus	E84.11	
277.Ø9	Cystic Fibrosis w/ Other Sx	E84.8	
277.Ø2	Cystic Fibrosis w/ Pulmonary Sx	E84.Ø+	*for any infectious organisms*
277.ØØ	Cystic Fibrosis w/o Meconium Ileus	E84.9	

3. Endocrine, Nutritional and Metabolic Diseases, and Immunity Disorders *(cont)*

ICD-9-CM		ICD-10-CM	
276.51	Dehydration	E86.0	excludes neonatal
		P74.1	neonatal
259.0	Delayed Puberty	E30.0	
249.00	Diabetes Mellitus, Secondary, Controlled	E09.-*+	Diabetes Mellitus, Due to Drug or Chemical *poisoning due to drug or toxin, T36–T65 for adverse effect, to identify drug T36–T50, and insulin use Z79.4*
		E08.-+	Diabetes Mellitus, Due to Underlying Condition *to identify condition and insulin use Z79.4*
249.01	Diabetes Mellitus, Secondary, Uncontrolled	E09.65	Diabetes Mellitus, Due to Drug or Chemical, w/ Hyperglycemia
		E09.641	Diabetes Mellitus, Due to Drug or Chemical, w/ Hypoglycemia w/ Coma
		E09.649	Diabetes Mellitus, Due to Drug or Chemical, w/ Hypoglycemia w/o Coma
		E08.65	Diabetes Mellitus, Due to Underlying Condition, w/ Hyperglycemia
		E08.641	Diabetes Mellitus, Due to Underlying Condition, w/ Hypoglycemia w/ Coma
		E08.649	Diabetes Mellitus, Due to Underlying Condition, w/ Hypoglycemia w/o Coma
250.01	Diabetes Mellitus Type 1, Controlled	E10.9	Diabetes Mellitus, Type 1, w/o Complications
250.03	Diabetes Mellitus Type 1, Uncontrolled	E10.9	Diabetes Mellitus, Type 1, w/o Complications
250.00	Diabetes Mellitus Type 2, Controlled	E11.9	Diabetes Mellitus, Type 2, w/o Complications
250.02	Diabetes Mellitus Type 2, Uncontrolled	E11.9	Diabetes Mellitus, Type 2, w/o Complications

ICD-9-CM		ICD-10-CM	
249.11	Diabetic Ketoacidosis, Secondary, Uncontrolled	E09.11	Diabetes Mellitus, Due to Drug or Chemical, w/ Ketoacidosis, w/ Coma
		E09.10	Diabetes Mellitus, Due to Drug or Chemical, w/ Ketoacidosis, w/o Coma
		E08.11	Diabetes Mellitus, Due to Underlying Condition, w/ Ketoacidosis, w/ Coma
		E08.10	Diabetes Mellitus, Due to Underlying Condition, w/ Ketoacidosis, w/o Coma
250.13	Diabetic Ketoacidosis Type 1, Uncontrolled	E10.11	w/ Coma
		E10.10	w/o Coma
279.11	DiGeorge Syndrome	D82.1	
259.4	Dwarfism, Endocrine	E34.3	
277.7	Dysmetabolic Syndrome X+	E88.81+	
276.9	*Electrolyte Imbalance*	E87.8	
277.85	Fatty Acid Oxidation Disorder Acyl Coenzyme A Dehydrogenase Deficiency Long-chain Acyl Coenzyme A Dehydrogenase Medium-chain Acyl Coenzyme A Dehydrogenase	E71.31-	
276.61	Fluid Overload Due to TACO	E87.71	
240.0	Goiter, Simple	E04.0	
279.51	Graft-vs-host Disease, Acute+	D89.810*+	*underlying cause, to identify manifestations*
279.53	Graft-vs-host Disease, Acute on Chronic+	D89.812*+	*underlying cause, to identify manifestations*
279.52	Graft-vs-host Disease, Chronic+	D89.811*+	*underlying cause, to identify manifestations*
271.0	G6PD Deficiency	D55.0	w/ Anemia
		E74.4	w/o Anemia
275.02	Hemochromatosis, Due to Repeated Transfusions	E83.111	
275.01	Hemochromatosis, Hereditary	E83.110	
275.42	Hypercalcemia	E83.52	

3. Endocrine, Nutritional and Metabolic Diseases, and Immunity Disorders *(cont)*

ICD-9-CM		ICD-10-CM	
272.0	Hypercholesterolemia	E78.0	
272.4	Hyperlipoproteinemia	E78.5	
276.0	Hypernatremia	E87.0	
242.90	Hyperthyroidism	E05.90	
273.8	Hypoalbuminemia	E88.09	
275.41	Hypocalcemia	E83.51	
279.00	Hypogammaglobulinemia	D80.1	
251.2	Hypoglycemia w/o Coma, Unspec	E16.2	
276.1	Hyponatremia	E87.1	
243	Hypothyroidism, Congenital	E03.1	
244.8	Hypothyroidism of Prematurity	E01.8	Iodine Deficiency
		E03.8	Other
244.9	Hypothyroidism, Unspec	E03.9	
276.52	Hypovolemia	E86.1	
279.3	Immunodeficiency, Unspec	D84.9	
277.9	Inborn Error of Metabolism, Unspec	E88.9	
271.3	Lactase Deficiency	E73.0	Congenital
		E73.1	Secondary
263.9	Malnutrition, Unspec	E46	
270.3	Maple Syrup Urine Disease	E71.0	
255.42	Mineralocorticoid Deficiency	E27.49	
	Hypoaldosteronism	E27.40	
277.87	Mitochondrial Metabolism Disorder	E88.4-	

ICD-9-CM		ICD-10-CM	
277.5	Mucopolysaccharide Disease	E76.3	Mucopolysaccharide Disease, Unspec
	Hunter Syndrome	E76.1	
	Hurler Syndrome	E76.01	
	Morquio-Brailsford Disease	E76.210	Morquio A Mucopolysaccharidoses
		E76.211	Morquio B Mucopolysaccharidoses
		E76.219	Morquio Mucopolysaccharidoses, Unspec
278.03	Obesity Hypoventilation Syndrome	E66.8	
	Pickwickian Syndrome	E66.2	
278.01	Obesity, Morbid	E66.01	
	add code for BMI if known	Z68.-	
278.00	Obesity, Unspec	E66.9	
	add code for BMI if known	Z68.-	
278.02	Overweight	E66.3	
	add code for BMI if known	Z68.-	
277.86	Peroxisomal Disorders	E71.5-	
270.1	Phenylketonuria	E70.0	Phenylketonuria, Classical
256.4	Polycystic Ovaries	E28.2	
259.1	Precocious Sexual Development	E30.1	
268.0	Rickets, Active	E55.0	
253.6	SIADH	E22.2	
240.9	Thyroid Enlargement	E01.2	Iodine Deficiency Related
		E004.9	Unspec
245.0	Thyroiditis, Acute	E06.0	
277.88	Tumor Lysis Syndrome	E88.3	
276.50	Volume Depletion, Unspec	E86.9	
279.12	Wiskott-Aldrich Syndrome	D82.0	
272.2	Xanthoma	E78.2	

3. Endocrine, Nutritional and Metabolic Diseases, and Immunity Disorders *(cont)*

ICD-9-CM		ICD-10-CM	
Other Related Diagnoses			
V21.8	Advanced Bone Age	Z00.2	
733.91	Arrested Bone Growth	M89.159	Femur
		M89.139	Forearm
		M89.129	Humerus
		M89.169	Lower Leg
		M89.18	Other Delayed Bone Age
V83.81	Carrier, Cystic Fibrosis Gene	Z14.1	
995.52	Child Neglect (Nutritional)	T74.02X√	Child Neglect, Confirmed
		T76.02X√	Child Neglect, Suspected
288.1	Chronic Granulomatous Disease	D71	
783.42	Delay in Developmental Milestones	R62.0	
783.40	Developmental Delay	R62.50	
775.1	Diabetes Mellitus, Neonatal	P70.2	
783.41	Failure to Thrive	R62.51	
779.34	Failure to Thrive in Newborn	P92.6	
783.3	Feeding Problem	R63.3	
779.31	Feeding Problems, Newborn	P92.8	
775.5	Fluid and Electrolyte Disturbances, Newborn	P74.4	
V26.33	Genetic Counseling	Z31.5	
791.5	Glycosuria	R81	
790.29	Hyperglycemia	R73.9	
775.4	Hypocalcemia, Newborn	P71.0	Cow's Milk Hypocalcemia
		P71.1	Other
775.6	Hypoglycemia, Newborn	P70.4	
790.22	Impaired Oral Glucose Tolerance Test	R73.02	
V58.67	Long-term (Current) Use of Insulin	Z79.4	
V58.65	Long-term (Current) Use of Steroids	Z79.51	Inhaled Steroids
		Z79.52	Systemic Steroids
579.8	*Milk/Formula Intolerance*	K90.4	

ICD-9-CM		ICD-10-CM	
796.6	Neonatal Screen, Nonspecific Abnormal Finding	PØ9	
V12.1	Nutritional Deficiency, Hx of	Z86.39	
V29.3	Obs for Genetic or Metabolic Condition, Newborn	PØØ.89	
783.9	*Other Sx Concerning Nutrition, Metabolism, and Development*	R63.8	Other Sx Food or Fluid Intake
783.5	Polydipsia/Excess Thirst	R63.1	
V21.1	Puberty	ZØØ.3	
V21.Ø	Rapid Growth in Childhood Accelerated Growth Rate	ZØØ.2	
V77.6	Screening for Cystic Fibrosis	Z13.228	
V77.1	Screening for Diabetes Mellitus	Z13.1	
V77.91	Screening for Lipid Disorders	Z13.22Ø	
783.43	Short Stature	R62.52	
V58.65	Steroids, Long-term (Current) Use	Z79.51	Inhaled Steroids
		Z79.52	Systemic Steroids
759.2	Thyroglossal Duct Cyst	Q89.2	
783.22	Underweight	R63.6	
	add code for BMI if known	Z68.-	
783.1	Weight Gain, Abnormal	R63.5	
783.21	Weight Loss, Abnormal	R63.4	
	add code for BMI if known	Z68.-	

4. Diseases of the Blood and Blood-forming Organs

ICD-10-CM codes are not valid for use at the time of publication and should not be reported until the official implementation date set by the Centers for Medicare & Medicaid Services.

ICD-9-CM		ICD-10-CM	
287.Ø	Allergic Purpura (Schönlein-Henoch)	D69.Ø	
285.9	*Anemia*	D64.9	
285.1	Anemia, Acute Blood Loss	D62	
285.3	Anemia, Antineoplastic Chemotherapy-Induced	D64.81	
282.2	Anemia, G6PD Deficiency	D55.Ø	
28Ø.1	Anemia, Iron Deficiency	D5Ø.8	
285.29	Anemia of Chronic Disease	D63.8*	
286.53	Antiphospholipid Antibody w/ Hemorrhagic Disorder	D68.312	
284.Ø1	Aplastic Anemia, Constitutional Blackfan-Diamond Syndrome	D61.Ø1	
284.89	Aplastic Anemia Due to Chronic Systemic Disease, Drugs, Infection§	D61.1	Due to Drugs
		D61.2	Due to Infection
		D61.89	Due to Chronic Systemic Disease
284.9	Aplastic Anemia, Unspec	D61.9	
288.66	Bandemia w/o Specific Infection Diagnosis	D72.825	
288.65	Basophilia	D72.824	
288.1	Chronic Granulomatous Disease	D71	
286.9	Coagulation Disorder	D68.9	
282.62	Dactylitis+	D57.ØØ	
286.6	DIC Syndrome	D65	
288.3	Eosinophilia	D72.1	
287.32	Evans Syndrome	D69.41	
284.Ø9	Fanconi Syndrome	D61.Ø9	
282.7	Hemoglobinopathy	D58.2	
	Hb-C Disease	D58.2	
	Hb-E Disease	D58.2	
	Persistent Fetal Hb	D56.4	

ICD-9-CM		ICD-10-CM	
288.4	Hemophagocytic Syndrome	D76.1	Hemophagocytic Lymphohistiocytosis Familial Hemophagocytic Reticulosis
		D76.2+	Hemophagocytic Syndrome, Infection-Associated *to identify infectious agent or disease*
		D76.3	Other Histiocytosis Syndromes Reticulohistiocytoma (Giant-Cell)
286.0	Hemophilia A (Factor VIII)	D66	
286.52	Hemophilia, Acquired	D68.311	
286.1	Hemophilia B (Factor IX)	D67	
286.59	Hemorrhagic Disorder, Due to Intrinsic Circulating Anticoagulants, Antibodies	D68.318	
287.31	Idiopathic Thrombocytopenic Purpura	D69.3	
288.62	Leukemoid Reaction	D72.823	
288.50	Leukocytopenia	D72.819	
288.60	Leukocytosis	D72.829	
289.3	Lymphadenitis	I88.9	
289.2	Lymphadenitis, Mesenteric	I88.0	
288.51	Lymphocytopenia	D72.810	
288.61	Lymphocytosis	D72.820	
289.7	Methemoglobinemia	D74.8	Acquired (Toxic)
		D74.0	Congenital
		D74.9	Unspec
288.63	Monocytosis (Symptomatic) Code 075 instead for Infectious Mononucleosis	D72.821	Code B27.- instead for Infectious Mononucleosis
284.2	Myelophthisis	D61.82+	*underlying disorder*

4. Diseases of the Blood and Blood-forming Organs *(cont)*

ICD-9-CM		ICD-10-CM	
288.01	Neutropenia, Congenital	D70.0	
	add 780.61 if fever present	R50.81	
288.02	Neutropenia, Cyclic	D70.4	
	add 780.61 if fever present	R50.81	
288.03	Neutropenia, Drug Induced§	D70.2	
288.04	Neutropenia, Due to Infection	D70.3	
	add 780.61 if fever present	R50.81	
288.09	Neutropenia, Other Immune Toxic	D70.8	
	add 780.61 if fever present	R50.81	
288.00	Neutropenia, Unspec	D70.9	
	add 780.61 if fever present	R50.81	
288.59	Other Decreased White Blood Cells	D72.818	
288.8	Other Specified White Blood Cell Disease	D72.89	
284.11	Pancytopenia, Antineoplastic Chemotherapy Induced	D61.810	
284.19	Pancytopenia, Other	D61.818	
284.12	Pancytopenia, Other Drug Induced	D61.811	
288.64	Plasmacytosis	D71.822	
289.0	Polycythemia	D75.1	
287.33	Purpura, Congenital and Hereditary Thrombocytopenic TAR Syndrome	D69.42*	*congenital or hereditary disorder such as TAR syndrome Q87.2*
287.31	Purpura, Immune Thrombocytopenic	D69.3	
287.41	Purpura, Posttransfusion	D69.51	
284.81	Red Cell Aplasia	D60.9	Red Cell Aplasia, Unspec

ICD-9-CM		ICD-10-CM	
282.60	Sickle Cell Disease, Unspec	D57.1	
282.64	Sickle Cell–Hb-C Disease w/ Crisis	D57.21±	
282.63	Sickle Cell–Hb-C Disease w/o Crisis	D57.20	
282.62	Sickle Cell–Hb-SS Disease w/ Crisis	D57.01	w/ Acute Chest Syndrome
		D57.02	w/ Splenic Sequestration
		D57.00	w/ Unspec Crisis
282.61	Sickle Cell–Hb-SS Disease w/o Crisis	D57.1	
282.69	Sickle Cell Other Type w/ Crisis	D57.81±	
282.68	Sickle Cell Other Type w/o Crisis	D57.80	
282.42	Sickle Cell–Thalassemia Disease w/ Crisis	D57.41±	
282.41	Sickle Cell–Thalassemia Disease w/o Crisis	D57.40±	
		±For Sickle Cell Codes, Use 6th Digit 1 w/ Acute Chest Syndrome; 2 w/ Splenic Sequestration; 9 for Unspec Crisis	
282.5	Sickle Cell Trait	D57.3	
282.0	Spherocytosis	D58.0	
289.52	Splenic Sequestration*	See Sickle Cell Above	
289.53	Splenomegaly, Neutropenic	D73.81	
282.43	Thalassemia, Alpha (Major) Hb-Bart Disease Hb-H Disease	D56.0	
282.44	Thalassemia, Beta (Major) Cooley Anemia Thalassemia Major	D56.1	
282.34	Thalassemia, Delta-Beta	D56.2	
282.47	Thalassemia, Hb-E-Beta	D56.5	
282.46	Thalassemia, Minor (Alpha/Beta) Thalassemia Trait	D56.3	
282.49	Thalassemia, Other w/o Sickle Cell Hb-C Thalassemia	D56.8	
282.40	Thalassemia, Unspec	D56.9	
287.39	Thrombocytopenia Primary, Other	D69.49	
287.49	Thrombocytopenia Secondary, Other	D69.59	
238.71	Thrombocytosis, Essential	D47.3	

4. Diseases of the Blood and Blood-forming Organs *(cont)*

ICD-9-CM		ICD-10-CM
Other Related Diagnoses		
776.6	Anemia of Prematurity	P61.2
V83.01	Carrier, Hemophilia A, Asymptomatic	Z14.01
V83.02	Carrier, Hemophilia A, Symptomatic	Z14.02
772.6	Cutaneous Hemorrhage, Newborn	P54.5
719.10	Hemarthrosis, Nontraumatic	M25.00
075	Infectious Mononucleosis	B27.-
204.00	Leukemia, Acute Lymphoid	C91.00
205.00	Leukemia, Acute Myeloid	C92.00
201.90	Lymphoma, Hodgkin	C81.90
V78.0	Screening for Iron Deficiency Anemia	Z13.0
V78.2	Screening for Sickle Cell	Z13.0
789.2	Splenomegaly	R16.1

5. Mental Cognitive Disorders

ICD-10-CM codes are not valid for use at the time of publication and should not be reported until the official implementation date set by the Centers for Medicare & Medicaid Services.

ICD-9-CM		ICD-10-CM	
313.83	Academic Underachievement	F93.8	
308.3	Acute Stress Reaction	F43.0	
314.01	ADD w/ Hyperactivity	F90.1	
314.00	ADD w/o Hyperactivity	F90.0	
309.22	Adjustment Disorder, Adolescent	F94.8	
309.21	Adjustment Disorder, Child/ Separation	F93.0	
309.89	Adjustment Disorder, Other	F43.29	
309.0	Adjustment Disorder w/ Depressed Mood Grief Reaction	F43.21	
309.82	Adjustment Disorder w/ Physical Sx	F43.8	
305.00	Alcohol Abuse	F10.10	Alcohol Abuse, Uncomplicated
303.90	Alcohol Dependence	F10.20	Alcohol Dependence, Uncomplicated
303.00	Alcohol Intoxication	F10.929	
305.70	Amphetamine Abuse	F15.10	
304.40	Amphetamine Dependence	F15.20	
307.1	Anorexia Nervosa	F50.00	
300.00	Anxiety	F41.9	
315.39	Articulation Development Disorder	F80.0	
299.80	Asperger Syndrome	F84.5	
299.00	Autistic Disorder, Current or Active	F84.0	
307.9	Behavior Activities Masturbation Nail Biting Thumb Sucking	F98.8	
307.51	Bulimia Nervosa	F50.2	
305.20	Cannabis Abuse	F12.10	Cannabis Abuse, Uncomplicated

5. **Mental Cognitive Disorders** *(cont)*

ICD-9-CM		ICD-10-CM	
305.60	Cocaine Abuse	F14.10	Cocaine Abuse, Uncomplicated
304.20	Cocaine Dependence	F14.20	Cocaine Dependence, Uncomplicated
312.82	Conduct Disorder, Adolescence	F91.2	
312.81	Conduct Disorder, Childhood	F91.1	
306.4	Cyclical Vomiting	F50.8	
311	Depression	F32.9	
296.20	Depression (Major), Acute	F32.9	
300.4	Depression w/ Anxiety	F41.8	Depression w/ Anxiety, Mild or Not Persistent
315.4	Developmental Coordination Disorder Clumsiness Syndrome	F82	
315.02	Developmental Dyslexia	F81.0	
315.39	Developmental Speech Delay	F80.0	
304.90	*Drug Dependence*	F19.29	
305.90	*Drug/Substance Abuse*	F19.19	
307.50	Eating Disorder, Atypical	F50.9	
307.7	Encopresis, Nonorganic	F98.1+	*identify cause of any coexisting constipation*
307.6	Enuresis, Nonorganic	F98.0	
307.59	Feeding Disorder of Infancy or Early Childhood	F98.29	
315.35	Fluency Disorder, Childhood Onset	F80.81	
307.81	Headaches, Tension	G44.209	
309.89	Homesickness	F43.8	
314.1	Hyperkinesis w/ Developmental Delay	F90.8	
314.2	Hyperkinetic Conduct Disorder	F90.8	
314.9	Hyperkinetic Syndrome	F90.9	
306.1	Hyperventilation, Psychogenic	F45.8	
300.7	Hypochondriasis	F45.22	

ICD-9-CM		ICD-10-CM	
300.11	Hysteria, Conversion Reaction	F44.4	Conversion Disorder w/ Motor Sx or Deficit
		F44.6	Conversion Disorder w/ Sensory Sx or Deficit
300.10	Hysterical Reaction	F44.9	
304.6	Inhalant Dependence	F18.20	Dependence
		F18.10	Abuse, Uncomplicated
317	Intellectual Disabilities, Mild, IQ 50–70	F70	
319	Intellectual Disabilities, Unspec	F79	
313.22	Introverted/Withdrawal Disorder	F93.8	
315.31	Language Disorder, Expressive	F80.1	
315.32	Language Disorder, Mixed Receptive-Expressive	F80.2	
	Central Auditory Processing Disorder	H93.25	
315.1	Learning Disorder, Mathematics	F81.2	
315.2	Learning Disorder, Other Specified	F81.89	
	Disorder of Written Expression	F81.81	
315.00	Learning Disorder, Reading	F81.0	
315.09	Learning Disorder, Spelling Difficulty	F81.81	
315.9	*Learning Disorder, Unspec*	F81.9	
305.20	Marijuana Abuse	F12.10	Marijuana Abuse, Uncomplicated
304.30	Marijuana Dependence	F12.20	Marijuana Dependence, Uncomplicated
313.1	*Misery/Unhappiness*	F93.8	
315.5	Mixed Development Disorder	F82	
307.46	Night Terrors	F51.4	
300.3	Obsessive-Compulsive Disorder	F42	
313.81	Oppositional Defiant Disorder	F91.3	
300.01	Panic Attack	F41.0	
301.9	Personality Disorder	F60.9	
304.60	Phencyclidine Dependence	F19.20	
300.20	Phobic Disorder	F40.9	

5. Mental Cognitive Disorders *(cont)*

ICD-9-CM		ICD-10-CM	
307.52	Pica	F98.3	
305.90	*Polysubstance Abuse*	F18.10	
304.80	Polysubstance Dependence	F19.20	
310.2	Post-concussion Syndrome	F07.81	
302.70	Psychosexual Dysfunction	R37	
302.6	Psychosexual Identity Disorder	F64.2	In Children
		F64.1	In Adolescence
299.90	Psychosis/Schizophrenia of Childhood	F84.9	
309.81	PTSD	F43.11	PTSD, Acute
		F43.12	PTSD, Chronic
		F43.10	PTSD, Unspec
307.3	Repetitive Movements Head Banging Spasmus Nutans	F98.4	
300.9	Self-mutilation	F48.9	
309.21	Separation Anxiety	F93.0	
302.9	Sexual Deviation	F65.9	
313.21	Shyness Disorder, Childhood	F94.8	
300.81	Somatization Disorder	F45.0	
315.34	Speech and Language Developmental Delay Due to Hearing Loss	F80.4*	*hearing loss H90.-, H91.-*
315.35	Stuttering	F80.81	
312.10	Temper Tantrums	F91.8	
307.21	Tic Disorder, Transient	F95.0	
307.20	Tic Disorder, Unspec	F95.9	
307.23	Tourette Syndrome	F95.2	

Other Related Diagnoses			
V61.41	Alcohol Abuse in Family	Z63.72	
V69.5	Behavioral Insomnia of Childhood	Z73.819	
V40.39	Behavioral Problems	F69	
995.51	Child Abuse, Emotional/ Psychological, Confirmed	T74.32X√	

ICD-9-CM		ICD-10-CM	
V61.10	Counsel Marital/Partner Problem	Z71.89	
V61.24	Counsel Parent-Adopted Child Problem	Z71.89	
V61.23	Counsel Parent-Biological Child Problem	Z71.89	
V61.25	Counsel Parent (Guardian)- Foster Child Problem	Z71.89	
V61.22	Counsel Perpetrator Parental Child Abuse	Z69.011	
V62.83	Counsel Perpetrator Sexual Abuse	Z69.82	
V61.12	Counsel Perpetrator Spousal Abuse	Z69.12	
V61.21	Counsel Victim Child Abuse	Z69.020	Counsel Victim Non-parental Child Abuse
		Z69.010	Counsel Victim Parental Child Abuse
V61.11	Counsel Victim Spousal Abuse	Z69.11	
783.42	Delay in Developmental Milestones	R62.0	
698.4	Dermatitis Factitia	L98.1	
783.40	Developmental Delay	R62.50	
784.61	Dyslexia	R48.0	
V62.3	Educational/Academic Problem	Z55.9	
V15.42	Emotional Abuse, Hx of	Z62.811	
V61.06	Family Disruption Due to Child in Foster Care or w/ Non-parental Family Member	Z63.32	
V61.05	Family Disruption Due to Child in Welfare Custody	Z63.32	
V61.07	Family Disruption Due to Death of Family Member	Z63.4	
V61.03	Family Disruption Due to Divorce or Legal Separation	Z63.5	
V61.01	Family Disruption Due to Family Member on Military Deployment	Z63.31	
V61.04	Family Disruption Due to Parent- Child Estrangement	Z63.8	
V61.02	Family Disruption Due to Return of Family Member From Military Deployment	Z63.8	
V61.09	Family Disruption, Other	Z63.8	

5. Mental Cognitive Disorders *(cont)*

ICD-9-CM		ICD-10-CM	
Other Related Diagnoses *(cont)*			
989.89	*Glue Sniffing*	T52.8X1√	Glue Sniffing, Accidental Poisoning
	E950.9 Intentional	T52.8X2√	Glue Sniffing, Intentional
V62.85	Homicidal Ideation	R45.85	
799.23	Impulsiveness	R45.87	
V40.0	Learning Problems	F81.9	
V65.2	Malingering	Z76.5	
V11.9	Mental Disorder, Hx of	Z86.59	
V71.02	Obs for Antisocial Behavior, Nonpsychiatric	Z03.89	
V71.09	Obs for Suspected Mental Condition	Z03.89	
V15.41	Physical Abuse, Hx of Child Physical/Sexual Abuse Rape	Z62.810	
V15.49	Psychological Trauma, Hx of	Z91.49	
780.50	Sleep Disturbance	G47.9	
N/A	Self-harm, Hx of	Z91.5	
V62.4	Social Maladjustment Cultural Deprivation	Z60.3	
784.59	Speech Disturbance	R47.89	
V61.42	Substance Abuse in Family	Z63.72	
V62.84	Suicide Attempt/Ideation/Risk	T14.91	Suicide Attempt
		R45.85	Suicide Ideation
V40.31	Wandering in Diseases Classified Elsewhere*	Z91.83*	

6. Diseases of the Nervous System and Sense Organs

ICD-10-CM codes are not valid for use at the time of publication and should not be reported until the official implementation date set by the Centers for Medicare & Medicaid Services.

ICD-9-CM		ICD-10-CM	
DISEASES OF THE NERVOUS SYSTEM			
348.1	Anoxic Brain Damage	G93.1	
351.8	Asymmetric Cry/Face	G51.8	
334.8	Ataxia-telangiectasia Louis-Bar Syndrome	G11.3	
351.0	Bell Palsy	G51.0	
333.1	Benign Myoclonus of Infancy	G25.3	
348.82	Brain Death	G93.82	
334.3	Cerebellar Ataxia	G11.1	Early-Onset Cerebellar Ataxia
		G11.2	Late-Onset Cerebellar Ataxia
330.9	Cerebral Degeneration, Childhood	G31.89	
348.5	Cerebral Edema	G93.6	
343.9	Cerebral Palsy, Infantile, Unspec	G80.9	
339.00	Cluster Headaches	G44.009	Cluster Headache Syndrome, Unspec, Not Intractable
323.61	Encephalitis, Infectious Acute Disseminated*	G04.00	
323.62	Encephalitis, Other Postinfectious*	G04.01	
323.51	Encephalitis, Postvaccination§	G04.02+	*identify the vaccine T50.A-, T50.B-, T50.Z-*
323.9	Encephalitis, Unspec	G04.90	
348.30	Encephalopathy, Unspec	G93.40	

6. Diseases of the Nervous System and Sense Organs *(cont)*

ICD-9-CM	ICD-10-CM
DISEASES OF THE NERVOUS SYSTEM *(cont)*	
345.10 Epilepsy, Generalized Convulsive Grand Mal Epilepsy Myoclonic Epilepsy	**G40.30±** Epilepsy, Generalized Idiopathic
345.11 Epilepsy, Generalized Convulsive, Poorly Controlled	**G40.31±** Epilepsy, Generalized, Idiopathic, Poorly Controlled
345.00 Epilepsy, Nonconvulsive Absence Seizures Petit Mal	**G40.A0±** Absence Epileptic Syndrome
	G40.A1± Absence Epileptic Syndrome, Poorly Controlled
	G40.30± Epilepsy, Generalized Idiopathic
	G40.B0± Juvenile Myoclonic Epilepsy (Impulsive Petit Mal)
	G40.B1± Juvenile Myoclonic Epilepsy (Impulsive Petit Mal), Poorly Controlled
345.01 Epilepsy, Nonconvulsive, Poorly Controlled	**G40.31±** Epilepsy, Generalized, Poorly Controlled
345.90 Epilepsy, Unspec (Seizure Disorder)	**G40.90±** Epilepsy, Unspec
345.91 Epilepsy, Unspec (Seizure Disorder), Poorly Controlled	**G40.91±** Epilepsy, Unspec, Poorly Controlled
	±For Epilepsy Codes, Use 6th Digit 1 for Status Epilepticus; 9 for w/o Status
334.0 Friedreich Ataxia	**G11.1**
357.0 Guillain-Barré Syndrome	**G61.0**
342.90 Hemiplegia	**G81.92** Unspec, Affecting Left Dominant Side
	G81.94 Unspec, Affecting Left Nondominant Side
	G81.91 Unspec, Affecting Right Dominant Side
	G81.93 Unspec, Affecting Right Nondominant Side
	G81.90 Unspec, Affecting Unspec Side

ICD-9-CM		ICD-10-CM	
342.00	Hemiplegia, Flaccid	G81.02	Flaccid Hemiplegia Affecting Left Dominant Side
		G81.04	Flaccid Hemiplegia Affecting Left Nondominant Side
		G81.01	Flaccid Hemiplegia Affecting Right Dominant Side
		G81.03	Flaccid Hemiplegia Affecting Right Nondominant Side
		G81.00	Flaccid Hemiplegia Affecting Unspec Side
342.10	Hemiplegia, Spastic	G81.12	Spastic Hemiplegia Affecting Left Dominant Side
		G81.14	Spastic Hemiplegia Affecting Left Nondominant Side
		G81.11	Spastic Hemiplegia Affecting Right Dominant Side
		G81.13	Spastic Hemiplegia Affecting Right Nondominant Side
		G81.10	Spastic Hemiplegia Affecting Unspec Side
327.22	High-altitude Periodic Breathing	G47.32	
331.3	Hydrocephalus, Communicating (Acquired)	G91.0	
331.5	Hydrocephalus, Idiopathic Normal Pressure	G91.2	
331.4	Hydrocephalus, Obstructive (Acquired)	G91.1	
345.60	Infantile Spasms/Hypsarrhythmia	G40.821	Epileptic Spasms, Not Intractable, w/ Status Epilepticus
		G40.822	w/o Status Epilepticus
		G40.823	Poorly Controlled, w/ Status Epilepticus
		G40.824	w/o Status Epilepticus
324.0	Intracranial Abscess	G06.0	

6. Diseases of the Nervous System and Sense Organs *(cont)*

ICD-9-CM		ICD-10-CM	
DISEASES OF THE NERVOUS SYSTEM *(cont)*			
320.9	Meningitis, Bacterial Unspec	G00.9	
320.82	Meningitis, Gram-negative	G00.9	
320.0	Meningitis, H. influenzae	G00.0	
320.1	Meningitis, Pneumococcal	G00.1	
320.2	Meningitis, Strep	G00.2+	*to identify organism* B95.0–B95.5
346.00	Migraine w/ Aura	G43.109	
346.02	Migraine w/ Aura w/ Status	G43.101	
346.10	Migraine w/o Aura	G43.009	
346.12	Migraine w/o Aura w/ Status	G43.001	
359.0	Muscular Dystrophy, Congenital	G71.0	
359.1	Muscular Dystrophy, Hereditary	G71.0	
358.01	Myasthenia Gravis w/ Exacerbation	G70.01	
358.00	Myasthenia Gravis w/o Exacerbation	G70.00	
323.63	Myelitis, Postinfectious*	G05.4	
323.52	Myelitis, Postvaccination§	G04.02+	*identify the vaccine* T50.A-, T50.B-, T50.Z-
333.2	Myoclonus Progressive Myoclonic Epilepsy	G25.3	
359.22	Myotonia, Congenital	G71.12	
358.9	*Neuromuscular Disorder*	G70.9	
338.11	Pain, Acute Due to Trauma	G89.11	
338.18	Pain, Acute, Postoperative	G89.18	
338.3	Pain, Neoplasm Related	G89.3	
338.19	Pain, Other Acute	R52	
344.9	Paralysis	G83.9	Paralytic Syndrome
344.1	Paraplegia	G82.21	Paraplegia, Complete
		G82.22	Paraplegia, Incomplete
		G82.20	Paraplegia, Unspec
346.20	Periodic Headache Syndrome	G43.C0	Not Intractable
346.22	Periodic Headache Syndrome w/ Status	G43.C1	Intractable
356.8	Peripheral Neuritis	G60.8	
345.2	Petit Mal Status	G40.301	
348.2	Pseudotumor Cerebri	G93.2	

ICD-9-CM		ICD-10-CM	
344.00	Quadriplegia	G82.50	
337.20	Reflex Sympathetic Dystrophy	G90.529	Complex Regional Pain Syndrome I of Unspec Lower Limb
		G90.519	Complex Regional Pain Syndrome I of Unspec Upper Limb
330.8	Rett Syndrome	F84.2	
345.90	Seizure Disorder	G40.901	w/ Status Epilepticus
		G40.909	w/o Status Epilepticus
345.91	Seizure Disorder, Poorly Controlled	G40.911	w/ Status Epilepticus
		G40.919	w/o Status Epilepticus
345.40	Seizures, Complex Partial (Partial w/ Impairment of Consciousness, Psychomotor)	G40.20±	Epilepsy, Localization-related Symptomatic w/ Complex Partial Seizures
345.41	Seizures, Complex Partial, Poorly Controlled	G40.21±	Epilepsy, Localization-related Symptomatic w/ Complex Partial Seizures, Poorly Controlled
345.50	Seizures, Simple Partial (Jacksonian Seizures, Partial, w/o Impairment of Consciousness)	G40.00±	Benign Childhood Epilepsy
		G40.10±	Epilepsy, Localization-related Symptomatic w/ Simple Partial Seizures
345.51	Seizures, Simple Partial, Poorly Controlled	G40.01±	Benign Childhood Epilepsy, Poorly Controlled
		G40.11±	Epilepsy, Localization-related Symptomatic w/ Simple Partial Seizures, Poorly Controlled
		±For Epilepsy Codes, Use 6th Digit 1 for Status Epilepticus; 9 for w/o Status	
327.23	Sleep Apnea, Obstructive	G47.33	
327.20	Sleep Apnea, Organic, Unspec	G47.30	
327.21	Sleep Apnea, Primary Central	G47.31	
330.1	Tay-Sachs Disease	E75.02	
348.81	Temporal Sclerosis	G93.81	
349.82	Toxic Encephalopathy§	G92*	to identify toxic agent T51–T65
335.0	Werdnig-Hoffmann Disease	G12.0	

6. **Diseases of the Nervous System and Sense Organs** (cont)

ICD-9-CM		ICD-10-CM	
DISEASES OF THE NERVOUS SYSTEM **Other Related Diagnoses**			
253.0	Acromegaly/Gigantism Sotos Syndrome	E22.0	
742.2	Agenesis Corpus Callosum	Q04.0	
305.00	Alcohol Abuse	F10.10	Alcohol Abuse, Uncomplicated
303.00	Alcohol Intoxication	F10.929	
780.97	Altered Mental Status	R41.82	
305.70	Amphetamine Abuse	F15.10	
756.0	Anomalies Skull/Face Megalocephaly/Large Head Premature Closure of the Sutures	Q75.8	
781.3	Ataxia	R27.0	
767.6	Brachial Plexus Injury, Newborn	P14.3	
	Erb Palsy	P14.0	
	Klumpke Palsy	P14.1	
V12.54	Cerebral Infarction w/o Residual Deficits (Intrauterine Stroke), Hx of	Z86.73	
851.80	*Cerebral Laceration and Contusion*	S06.330√	w/o LOC
V45.2	Cerebral VP/VA Shunt Present	Z98.2	
V12.42	CNS Infection, Hx of	Z86.61	
305.60	Cocaine Abuse	F14.10	Cocaine Abuse, Uncomplicated
780.01	Coma	R40.20	Coma, Unspec
850.5	Concussion w/ LOC, Unspec Duration	S06.0X9√	
850.0	Concussion w/o LOC	S06.0X0√	
742.9	Congenital Anomaly, CN	SQ07.9	
779.0	Convulsions, Newborn	P90	
783.42	Delay in Developmental Milestones	R62.0	
783.40	Developmental Delay	R62.50	
V49.85	Dual Sensory Impairment Combined Visual-Hearing Impairment	Z73.82	

ICD-9-CM		ICD-10-CM	
049.9	*Encephalitis, Viral*	A86	Encephalitis, Viral, Unspec
348.89	Encephalomalacia	G93.89	
780.1	Hallucinations	R44.0	Auditory
		R44.2	Other
		R44.3	Unspec
		R44.1	Visual
959.01	Head Injury w/o LOC	S09.8XX√	Head Injury, Other Specified
		S09.90X√	Head Injury, Unspec
784.0	Headache	R51	
307.81	Headaches, Tension	G44.209	
742.3	Hydrocephalus, Congenital	Q03.0	Malformations of Aqueduct of Sylvius
	Dandy-Walker Cyst	Q03.1	
		Q03.8	Other
		Q03.9	Unspec
437.2	Hypertensive Encephalopathy	I67.4	
431	Intracerebral Hemorrhage	I61.9	
432.9	Intracranial Hemorrhage, Nontraumatic	I62.9	
853.00	*Intracranial Hemorrhage, Traumatic*	S06.360√	w/o LOC
984.9	Lead Poisoning	T56.0X1√	Lead Poisoning, Accidental
	E866.0 Accidental		
790.6	Lead Test, Positive, Nonspecific	R78.71	
996.2	Malfunction CNS Shunt	T85.09X√	
305.20	Marijuana Abuse	F12.10	Marijuana Abuse, Uncomplicated
191.6	Medulloblastoma	C71.6	
036.0	Meningitis, Meningococcal	A39.0	
047.9	*Meningitis, Viral/Aseptic*	A87.9	Meningitis, Viral, Unspec
		G03.0	Meningitis, Aseptic
742.1	Microcephalus, Congenital	Q02	
V48.6	Molded Head	R68.89	
741.93	Myelomeningocele, Lumbar	Q05.7	
191.5	Neoplasm Brain Ventricle	C71.5	

6. Diseases of the Nervous System and Sense Organs *(cont)*

ICD-9-CM		ICD-10-CM	
DISEASES OF THE NERVOUS SYSTEM **Other Related Diagnoses** *(cont)*			
781.99	*Neurologic Complaints/Sx*	R29.90	
V12.49	Neurologic Disorder, Hx of	Z86.69	
V29.1	Obs for Suspected CNS Disease, Newborn Evaluation for Neonatal Seizure	P00.89	
989.3	Organophosphate Poison+	T60.0X4√	Organophosphate Poison, Undetermined
	E863.1 Accidental	T60.0X1√	
	E950.6 Intentional	T60.0X2√	
780.03	Persistent Vegetative State	R40.3	
305.9	Polysubstance Abuse	F18.10	
742.4	Porencephalic Cyst	Q04.6	excludes acquired
307.3	Repetitive Movements Head Banging Spasmus Nutans	F98.4	
780.39	Seizure/Convulsions	R56.9	
780.32	Seizure, Febrile, Complex	R56.01	
780.31	Seizure, Febrile, Simple	R56.00	
780.33	Seizure, Post-traumatic	R56.1	
995.55	Shaken Baby Syndrome	T74.4XX√	
741.00	Spina Bifida w/ Hydrocephalus	Q05.4	
	Arnold-Chiari Syndrome Type II	Q07.03	
741.90	Spina Bifida w/o Hydrocephalus	Q05.8	
952.9	*Spinal Cord Injury*	S14.109√	Cervical
		S34.109√	Lumbar
		S34.139√	Sacrum
		S24.109√	Thoracic
430	Subarachnoid Bleed, Nontraumatic	I60.9	
852.00	*Subarachnoid Bleed, Traumatic*	S06.6X9√	w/ LOC Unspec Duration
		S06.6X0√	w/o LOC
432.1	Subdural Hemorrhage, Nontraumatic	I62.9	
852.20	*Subdural Hemorrhage, Traumatic*	S06.5X9√	w/ LOC Unspec Duration
		S06.5X0√	w/o LOC

ICD-9-CM		ICD-10-CM	
780.2	Syncope/Fainting	R55	
307.21	Tic Disorder, Transient	F95.0	
307.20	Tic Disorder, Unspec	F95.9	
435.9	Transient Ischemic Attack	G45.9	
780.09	Unconsciousness/Stupor	R40.1	
989.5	Venomous Bite	T63.91X√	Venomous Bite, Unspec Animal, Accidental
	Bee	T63.441√	Accidental
	Jellyfish	T63.621√	Accidental
	Snake	T63.001√	Snake, Unspec, Accidental
	Spider	T63.301√	Spider, Unspec, Accidental
	Tick	T63.481√	Accidental

DISEASES OF THE EYE

ICD-9-CM		ICD-10-CM	
373.00	Blepharitis	H01.00-	
372.20	Blepharoconjunctivitis	H10.5¤	
368.8	Blurred Vision	H53.8	
366.00	Cataract, Infantile/Juvenile, Unspec	H26.00¤	
373.2	Chalazion/Meibomian Cyst	H00.1-	
372.73	Chemosis/Conjunctival Edema	H11.42¤	
372.72	Conjunctival/Sclera Hemorrhage	H11.3▲	
372.00	Conjunctivitis, Acute	H10.3▲	
372.06	Conjunctivitis, Acute Chemical	H10.21¤	
372.05	Conjunctivitis, Allergic	H10.1▲	
371.82	Contact Lens Irritation/Injury	H18.82¤	
375.30	Dacryocystitis, Acute	H40.3▲√	to define stage
378.00	*Esotropia*	H50.00	
378.10	*Exotropia*	H50.10	
374.84	Eyelid Cyst	H02.82-	
365.14	Glaucoma of Childhood	Q15.0	
373.11	Hordeolum (Stye)	H00.01-	by site

6. Diseases of the Nervous System and Sense Organs *(cont)*

ICD-9-CM		ICD-10-CM
DISEASES OF THE EYE *(cont)*		
362.70	Macula Degeneration, Hereditary	H35.50
352.6	Möbius Syndrome	G52.7
375.55	Nasolacrimal Duct Obstruction, Newborn	H04.53¤
379.50	*Nystagmus*	H55.00
377.43	Optic Nerve Hypoplasia	H47.03¤
376.01	Orbital Cellulitis	H05.01¤
377.00	*Papilledema*	H47.10
373.13	Periorbital Cellulitis	H00.03-
376.00	Preseptal Cellulitis	H05.00
374.30	Ptosis, Acquired	H02.40¤
367.9	*Refractive Error*	H52.7
362.75	Retinal Cone Dystrophy	H35.53
362.22	Retinopathy of Prematurity, Stage 0	H35.11¤
362.23	Retinopathy of Prematurity, Stage 1	H35.12¤
362.24	Retinopathy of Prematurity, Stage 2	H35.13¤
362.25	Retinopathy of Prematurity, Stage 3	H35.14¤
362.26	Retinopathy of Prematurity, Stage 4	H35.15¤
362.27	Retinopathy of Prematurity, Stage 5	H35.16¤
362.20	Retinopathy of Prematurity, Unspec	H35.10¤
362.21	Retrolental Fibroplasia	H35.17¤
378.9	*Strabismus*	H50.9
368.9	*Visual Disturbance*	H53.9
369.9	*Visual Impairment*	H54.7

ICD-9-CM		ICD-10-CM	
Other Related Diagnoses			
743.30	Cataract, Congenital, Unspec	Q12.0	
743.46	Coloboma Iris	Q13.0	
743.9	*Congenital Anomaly, Eye*	Q15.9	
077.98	Conjunctivitis, Chlamydia	A74.89	excludes neonatal
		P39.1	neonatal
771.6	Conjunctivitis/Dacryocystitis, Newborn	P39.1	
098.40	Conjunctivitis, Gonococcal, Newborn	A54.31	
077.99	Conjunctivitis, Viral	B30.9	
918.1	Corneal Abrasion	S05.02X√	Left Eye
		S05.01X√	Right Eye
		S05.00X√	Unspec Eye
930.1	Foreign Body, Conjunctiva	T15.12X√	Left Eye
		T15.11X√	Right Eye
		T15.10X√	Unspec Eye
930.0	Foreign Body, Corneal	T15.02X√	Left Eye
		T15.01X√	Right Eye
		T15.00X√	Unspec Eye
802.6	Fx Orbit (Blowout), Closed	S02.3XX√	
743.20	Glaucoma, Congenital	Q15.0	
870.1	Laceration, Eyelid	S01.11X√	
743.61	Ptosis, Congenital	Q10.0	
V72.0	Vision Exam, Special not part of a routine or general exam	Z01.01	Vision Exam w/ Abnormal Findings
		Z01.00	Vision Exam w/o Abnormal Findings
V41.0	Visual Impairment Problem	H54.7	

6. Diseases of the Nervous System and Sense Organs *(cont)*

ICD-9-CM		ICD-10-CM	
DISEASES OF THE EAR			
384.01	Bullous Myringitis	H73.01¤	
380.4	Cerumen, Impacted (Earwax)	H61.2▲	
381.81	Eustachian Tube Dysfunction	H69.9▲	
389.14	Hearing Loss, Central	H90.5	
389.06	Hearing Loss, Conductive Bilateral	H90.0	
389.05	Hearing Loss, Conductive Unilateral	H90.12	Left Ear
		H90.11	Right Ear
389.00	Hearing Loss, Conductive Unspec	H90.2	
389.22	Hearing Loss, Mixed Bilateral	H90.6	
389.21	Hearing Loss, Mixed Unilateral	H90.72	Left Ear
		H90.71	Right Ear
389.20	Hearing Loss, Mixed Unspec	H90.8	
389.13	Hearing Loss, Neural Unilateral	H90.42	Left Ear
		H90.41	Right Ear
389.18	Hearing Loss, Sensorineural Bilateral	H90.3	
389.10	Hearing Loss, Sensorineural Unspec	H90.5	
389.17	Hearing Loss, Sensory Unilateral	H90.42	Left Ear
		H90.41	Right Ear
389.9	*Impairment of Hearing*	H91.9▲	
386.30	Labyrinthitis	H83.0¤	
388.70	*Otalgia (Earache)*	H92.0¤	
380.10	Otitis Externa	H60.9▲	
381.01	Otitis Media, Acute, Serous	H65.0▲	
		H66.06	Recurrent, Bilateral
		H66.05	Recurrent, Left
		H66.04	Recurrent, Right
		H66.07	Recurrent, Unspec

ICD-9-CM		ICD-10-CM
382.00	Otitis Media, Acute, Suppurative (Purulent)	H66.00¤
		H66.006 Recurrent, Bilateral
		H66.005 Recurrent, Left
		H66.004 Recurrent, Right
		H66.007 Recurrent, Unspec
382.02	Otitis Media, Acute, Suppurative (Purulent) w/ Associated Condition*	H67.¤*+ *code first underlying disease, perforated tympanic membrane H72.-*
382.01	Otitis Media, Acute, Suppurative (Purulent) w/ Rupture	H66.01¤
		H66.016 Recurrent, Bilateral
		H66.015 Recurrent, Left
		H66.014 Recurrent, Right
		H66.017 Recurrent, Unspec
382.3	Otitis Media, Chronic, Suppurative (Purulent)	H66.3X¤
381.10	Otitis Media, Chronic, Serous	H65.2▲
381.4	Otitis Media w/ Effusion	H65.9▲
388.60	Otorrhea (Non-CSF)	H92.1▲
384.20	Perforated Eardrum, Nontraumatic	H72.9▲
380.12	Swimmer's Ear	H60.33¤
388.30	Tinnitus	H93.1¤

Other Related Diagnoses		
744.3	*Congenital Anomaly, Ear*	Q17.9
931	Foreign Body, Ear	T16.2XX√ in Left Ear
		T16.1XX√ in Right Ear
		T16.9XX√ in Unspec Ear
V72.12	Hearing Conservation and Treatment	Z01.12
V72.11	Hearing Exam After Failed Hearing Screen	Z01.110
V41.2	Hearing Problem	H93.299

6. Diseases of the Nervous System and Sense Organs *(cont)*

ICD-9-CM	ICD-10-CM
DISEASES OF THE EAR **Other Related Diagnoses** *(cont)*	
872.00 Laceration, Ears	**S01.312√** Laceration w/o Foreign Body of Left Ear
	S01.311√ Laceration w/o Foreign Body of Right Ear
	S01.319√ Laceration w/o Foreign Body, Unspec Ear
994.6 Motion Sickness	**T75.3XX√** *identify vehicle or type of motion Y92.81-, Y93.5-*
872.61 Perforated Eardrum, Traumatic	**S09.22X√** Traumatic Rupture of Left Eardrum
	S09.21X√ Traumatic Rupture of Right Eardrum
	S09.20X√ Traumatic Rupture of Unspec Eardrum
780.4 Vertigo (Dizziness)	**R42**

7. Diseases of the Circulatory System

ICD-10-CM codes are not valid for use at the time of publication and should not be reported until the official implementation date set by the Centers for Medicare & Medicaid Services.

ICD-9-CM		ICD-10-CM	
443.89	Acrocyanosis	I73.89	
427.9	*Arrhythmia, Cardiac*	I49.9	
427.89	Bradycardia, Sinus	RØØ.1	
423.3	Cardiac Tamponade*	I31.4*	
429.3	Cardiomegaly	I51.7	
425.18	Cardiomyopathy, Hypertrophic Nonobstructive	I42.2	
425.11	Cardiomyopathy, Hypertrophic Obstructive	I42.1	
425.4	Cardiomyopathy, Primary	I42.5	
425.9	Cardiomyopathy, Secondary	I42.9	
427.5	Cardiorespiratory Arrest	I46.9	Cause Unspec
		I46.2	Due to Underlying Cardiac Condition
		I46.8*	Due to Other Underlying Condition *underlying condition*
459.9	*Cardiovascular Disease, Unspec*	I99.9	
426.9	*Conduction Disorder*	I45.9	
428.Ø	Congestive Heart Failure	I5Ø.9	
348.89	Encephalomalacia	G93.89	
421.9	Endocarditis, Acute	I33.9	
421.Ø	Endocarditis, Acute Bacterial	I33.Ø	
455.6	Hemorrhoids	K64.-	
455.8	Hemorrhoids, Bleeding	K64.-	
4Ø1.9	Hypertension, Essential	I1Ø	
437.2	Hypertensive Encephalopathy	I67.4	
458.9	Hypotension	I95.9	
458.Ø	Hypotension, Orthostatic	I95.1	
431	Intracerebral Hemorrhage	I61.9	
432.9	Intracranial Hemorrhage, Nontraumatic	I62.9	
446.1	Kawasaki Disease/MCLS	M3Ø.3	
426.82	Long QT Syndrome	I45.81	

7. Diseases of the Circulatory System *(cont)*

ICD-9-CM		ICD-10-CM	
425.8	Marfan Cardiomyopathy code Marfan Syndrome (759.82) first	Q87.418£	Marfan Syndrome w/ Other Cardiomyopathy
424.0	Mitral Valve Prolapse	I34.0	
422.90	Myocarditis, Acute	I40.9	
420.99	Pericarditis, Acute Purulent	I30.8	
420.91	Pericarditis, Acute Viral	I30.0+	to identify infectious agent B95–B97
451.9	*Phlebitis*	I80.9	
453.3	Renal Vein Thrombosis	I82.3	
390	Rheumatic Fever, Acute	I00	
391.9	*Rheumatic Heart Disease*	I01.9	
430	Subarachnoid Bleed, Nontraumatic	I60.9	
432.1	Subdural Hemorrhage, Nontraumatic	I62.00	
427.0	Supraventricular Tachycardia	I47.1	
435.9	Transient Ischemic Attack	G45.9	
456.4	Varicocele	I86.1	
426.7	Wolff-Parkinson-White Syndrome	I45.6	

Other Related Diagnoses			
995.0	Anaphylactic Shock/Reaction	T78.2XX√
746.3	Aortic Stenosis	Q23.0
745.5	Atrial Septal Defect	Q21.1
745.69	Atrioventricular Canal	Q21.2
779.81	Bradycardia, Newborn	P29.12
779.85	Cardiac Arrest of Newborn	P29.81
V45.01	Cardiac Pacemaker Present	Z95.0
785.9	*Cardiovascular Complaints/Sx*	R09.89
V15.1	Cardiovascular Surgery, Hx of	Z98.89
786.50	Chest Pain	R07.9
747.10	Coarctation of Aorta	Q25.1
746.9	*Congenital Heart Disease, Unspec*	Q24.9
782.5	Cyanosis	R23.0

ICD-9-CM		ICD-10-CM	
796.2	*Elevated BP, w/o Hypertension*	R03.0	
745.60	Endocardial Cushion Defect	Q21.2	
747.83	Fetal Circulation, Persistent	P29.3	
763.83	*Fetal Heart Rate/Rhythm Abnormality*	P03.810	Onset Before Labor
		P03.811	Onset During Labor
		P03.819	Unspec Time of Onset
V42.1	Heart Transplant Present	Z94.1	
V43.3	Heart Valve Present, Prosthesis	Z95.2	
V42.2	Heart Valve Present, Transplant	Z95.3	
746.7	Hypoplastic Left Heart	Q23.4	
V58.66	Long-term (Current) Use of Aspirin	Z79.82	
785.2	Murmur, Undiagnosed Condition not to be used for functional murmur	R01.0	Murmur, Benign and Innocent (Functional)
		R01.1	Murmur, Heart NOS
785.1	Palpitations	R00.2	
747.0	Patent Ductus Arteriosus	Q25.0	
747.32	Pulmonary Arteriovenous Malformation	Q25.72	
747.39	Pulmonary Artery Anomalies	Q25.79	
747.31	Pulmonary Artery Coarctation and Atresia	Q25.5	Pulmonary Artery Atresia
		Q25.71	Pulmonary Artery Coarctation
746.02	Pulmonary Valve Stenosis	Q22.1	
785.51	Shock, Cardiogenic	R57.0	
785.50	Shock, Nontraumatic	R57.9	
785.52	Shock, Septic add 995.92 if organ dysfunction present	R65.21*	Sepsis, Severe, w/ Septic Shock
958.4	Shock, Traumatic	T79.4XX√	
V12.53	Sudden Cardiac Arrest, Hx of	Z86.74	
V17.41	Sudden Cardiac Death, Family Hx of	Z82.41	
785.0	Tachycardia	R00.0	
779.82	Tachycardia, Newborn	P29.11	
745.2	Tetralogy of Fallot	Q21.3	

7. Diseases of the Circulatory System *(cont)*

ICD-9-CM		ICD-10-CM
Other Related Diagnoses *(cont)*		
747.41	Total Anomalous Pulmonary Venous Return	Q26.2
745.1Ø	Transposition of Great Vessels	Q2Ø.3
745.Ø	Truncus Arteriosus	Q2Ø.Ø
212.7	Tumor, Benign, Heart	D15.1
745.4	Ventricular Septal Defect	Q21.Ø

8. Diseases of the Respiratory System

ICD-10-CM codes are not valid for use at the time of publication and should not be reported until the official implementation date set by the Centers for Medicare & Medicaid Services.

ICD-9-CM		ICD-10-CM
DISEASES OF THE THROAT AND SINUS		
477.2	Allergic Rhinitis Due to Animal Hair	J30.81
477.8	Allergic Rhinitis Due to Dust	J30.89
477.1	Allergic Rhinitis Due to Food	J30.5
477.0	Allergic Rhinitis Due to Pollen	J30.1
478.6	Edema Subglottic/Glottis	J38.4
464.31	Epiglottitis, Acute w/ Obstruction	J05.11
464.30	Epiglottitis, Acute w/o Obstruction	J05.10
474.12	Hypertrophy of Adenoids	J35.2
474.11	Hypertrophy of Tonsils	J35.1
474.10	Hypertrophy of Tonsils and Adenoids	J35.8
464.01	Laryngitis, Acute w/ Obstruction	J05.0
464.00	Laryngitis, Acute w/o Obstruction	J04.0
464.21	Laryngotracheitis, Acute w/ Obstruction	J05.0
464.20	Laryngotracheitis, Acute w/o Obstruction	J04.2
471.0	Nasal Polyps	J33.0
470	Nasal Septum Deviation	J34.2
460	Nasopharyngitis, Acute/Common Cold	J00
475	Peritonsillar Abscess	J36
462	Pharyngitis, Acute/Sore Throat	J02.9
478.24	Retropharyngeal Abscess	J39.0
472.0	Rhinitis, Chronic, Nonallergic	J31.0
461.9	*Sinusitis, Acute, Unspec Site*	J01.90
473.9	*Sinusitis, Chronic*	J32.9
461.0	Sinusitis, Maxillary, Acute	J01.00
472.1	Sore Throat, Chronic	J31.2
464.51	Supraglottitis, w/ Obstruction	J04.31
464.50	Supraglottitis, w/o Obstruction	J04.30
463	Tonsillitis, Acute	J03
474.00	Tonsillitis, Chronic	J35.0

8. Diseases of the Respiratory System (cont)

ICD-9-CM		ICD-10-CM	
DISEASES OF THE THROAT AND SINUS (cont)			
464.11	Tracheitis, Acute w/ Obstruction	J04.11	
464.10	Tracheitis, Acute w/o Obstruction	J04.10	
465.9	URI, Acute	J06.9	

Other Related Diagnoses			
V15.09	Allergic to Other Nonmedicinal Agents	Z91.048	
V15.03	Allergy to Eggs	Z91.012	
V15.02	Allergy to Milk	Z91.011	
V15.05	Allergy to Other Foods	Z91.018	
V15.01	Allergy to Peanuts	Z91.010	
749.10	*Cleft Lip*	Q36.0	Bilateral
		Q36.1	Median
		Q36.9	Unilateral (NOS)
749.00	*Cleft Palate*	Q35.1	Cleft Hard Palate
		Q35.5	Cleft Hard Palate w/Cleft Soft Palate
		Q35.9	Cleft Palate, Unspec
		Q35.3	Cleft Soft Palate
784.7	Epistaxis/Nosebleed	R04.0	
932	Foreign Body, Nose	T17.1XX√	
802.0	Fx Nasal Bone, Closed	S02.2XX√	
784.42	Hoarseness	R49.0	
873.20	Laceration, Nose	S01.21X√	
748.0	Nasal Stenosis/Choanal Atresia	Q30.0	
528.3	Oral Cellulitis and Abscess	K12.2	
784.91	Postnasal Drip	R09.82	
034.0	Strep Sore Throat	J02.0	Strep Pharyngitis/Sore Throat
		J03.00	Strep Tonsillitis, Acute
		J03.01	Strep Tonsillitis, Recurrent
784.99	*Throat/Mouth Complaints/Sx*	R06.89	
	Halitosis	R19.6	
	Mouth Breathing	R06.5	
784.1	Throat Pain	R07.0	

ICD-9-CM		ICD-10-CM	
DISEASES OF THE RESPIRATORY SYSTEM			
517.3	Acute Chest Syndrome*	J99*	*underlying disease*
512.84	Air Leak, Persistent	J93.82	
512.2	Air Leak, Postoperative	J95.812	
516.64	Alveolar Capillary Dysplasia w/ Vein Misalignment	J84.843	
493.02 493.12 493.92	Asthma, Extrinsic, w/ Acute Exacerbation Asthma, Intrinsic, w/ Acute Exacerbation *Asthma, Unspec, w/ Acute Exacerbation*	J45.21 J45.31 J45.41 J45.51 J45.901	Asthma w/ Acute Exacerbation, Mild Intermittent Asthma, w/ Acute Exacerbation, Mild Persistent Asthma, w/ Acute Exacerbation, Moderate Persistent Asthma, w/ Acute Exacerbation, Severe Persistent Asthma, w/ Acute Exacerbation, Unspec
493.01 493.11 493.91	Asthma, Extrinsic, w/ Status Asthma, Intrinsic, w/ Status Asthma, Unspec, w/ Status	J45.22 J45.32 J45.42 J45.52 J45.902	Asthma, w/ Status, Mild Intermittent Asthma, w/ Status, Mild Persistent Asthma, w/ Status, Moderate Persistent Asthma, w/ Status, Severe Persistent Asthma, w/ Status, Unspec
493.00 493.10 493.90	Asthma, Extrinsic, Unspec Asthma, Intrinsic, Unspec *Asthma, Unspec, Unspec*	J45.20 J45.30 J45.40 J45.50 J45.909	Asthma, Unspec, Mild Intermittent Asthma, Unspec, Mild Persistent Asthma, Unspec, Moderate Persistent Asthma, Unspec, Severe Persistent Asthma, Unspec, Uncomplicated (Asthma, NOS)
488.01	Avian Flu	J09.X1	

8. Diseases of the Respiratory System *(cont)*

ICD-9-CM		ICD-10-CM
DISEASES OF THE RESPIRATORY SYSTEM *(cont)*		
466.19	Bronchiolitis, Due to Other Organisms	J21.8
466.11	Bronchiolitis, RSV	J21.Ø
466.Ø	Bronchitis, Acute	J2Ø.9
485	Bronchopneumonia	J18.Ø
519.11	Bronchospasm, Acute	J98.Ø1
493.82	Cough Variant Asthma	J45.991
464.4	Croup	JØ5.Ø
493.81	Exercised-induced Bronchospasm	J45.99Ø
488.82	Influenza, Novel A	JØ9.X2
488.89	Influenza, Novel A w/ Other Manifestations	JØ9.X9
488.81	Influenza, Novel A w/ Pneumonia	JØ9.X1
487.1	Influenza, Seasonal	J11.1
487.8	Influenza, Seasonal w/ Other Manifestations	J11.89+ *manifestations*
487.Ø	Influenza, Seasonal w/ Pneumonia	J11.ØØ
488.19	Influenza, 2ØØ9 H1N1 w/ Other Manifestations	JØ9.X9
488.12	Influenza, 2ØØ9 H1N1 w/ Other Respiratory Manifestations	JØ9.X2
488.11	Influenza, 2ØØ9 H1N1 w/ Pneumonia	JØ9.X1
516.69	Interstitial Lung Disease of Childhood	J84.848
518.1	Mediastinal Air/ Pneumomediastinum	J98.2
516.61	Neuroendocrine Cell Hyperplasia of Infancy	J84.841
519.4	Paralysis of Diaphragm	J98.6
511.9	Pleural Effusion	J9Ø
511.Ø	Pleurisy	RØ9.1
5Ø7.Ø	Pneumonia, Aspiration	J69.Ø+ *any associated foreign body in respiratory tract T17.-*
482.9	Pneumonia, Bacterial	J15.9
483.1	Pneumonia, Chlamydial	J16.Ø

ICD-9-CM		ICD-10-CM	
516.8	Pneumonia, Interstitial	J84.09	
507.1	Pneumonia, Lipoid	J69.1*	*to identify substance T51–T65*
482.42	Pneumonia, MRSA	J15.212	
482.41	Pneumonia, MSSA	J15.211	
483.0	Pneumonia, Mycoplasma	J15.7	
486	Pneumonia, Organism Unspec Atypical	J18.9	
481	Pneumonia, Pneumococcal (Lobar)	J18.1	
480.9	Pneumonia, Viral	J12.9	
512.89	Pneumothorax	J93.9	
512.83	Pneumothorax, Chronic	J93.81	
512.81	Pneumothorax, Spontaneous Primary	J93.11	
512.82	Pneumothorax, Spontaneous Secondary	J93.12*	*underlying condition*
512.0	Pneumothorax, Spontaneous Tension	J93.0	
516.62	Pulmonary Interstitial Glycogenosis	J84.842	
493.90	*Reactive Airway Disease*	J45.909	
493.92	*Reactive Airway Disease, Acute Exacerbation*	J45.901	
508.2	Respiratory Condition From Smoke Inhalation+§	J70.5	
518.81	Respiratory Failure, Acute	J96.81	
518.84	Respiratory Failure, Acute and Chronic	J96.20	
518.51	Respiratory Failure, Acute Following Trauma or Surgery	J95.821	Postprocedural
	ARDS Related to Trauma or Surgery	J96.00	Trauma
518.83	Respiratory Failure, Chronic	J96.10	
518.82	Respiratory Insufficiency, Acute	J80	
516.63	Surfactant Mutations of the Lung	J84.83	
518.7	TRALI	J95.84	

8. Diseases of the Respiratory System *(cont)*

ICD-9-CM		ICD-10-CM	
DISEASES OF THE RESPIRATORY SYSTEM **Other Related Diagnoses**			
786.7	Abnormal Chest Sounds (Not Wheezing) Rales Rhonchi	R09.89	
786.03	Apnea	R06.81	
770.82	Apnea, Newborn, Other	R28.4	
770.81	Apnea, Primary of Newborn	R28.3	
799.01	Asphyxia	R09.01	
994.7	Asphyxiation/Strangulation	T71.9XX√	
770.7	Bronchopulmonary Dysplasia	P27.1	
986	Carbon Monoxide Inhalation	T58.94X√	Unspec Source, Undetermined
	E868.8 Accidental	T58.91X√	Unspec Source
	E952.1 Intentional	T58.92X√	Unspec Source
786.04	Cheyne-Stokes Respiration	R06.3	
748.9	*Congenital Anomaly, Respiratory*	Q34.9	
786.2	Cough	R05	
782.5	Cyanosis	R23.0	
770.83	Cyanosis, Newborn	P28.2	
277.02	Cystic Fibrosis w/ Pulmonary Sx	E84.0+	*for any infectious organisms*
994.1	Drowning, Fatal or Nonfatal	T75.1XX√	
770.16	Fetal and Newborn Aspiration of Blood w/ Respiratory Sx	P24.21	
770.14	Fetal and Newborn Aspiration of Clear Amniotic Fluid w/ Respiratory Sx	P24.11	
770.86	Fetal and Newborn Aspiration of Postnatal Stomach Contents w/ Respiratory Sx	P24.31	
770.18	Fetal and Newborn Aspiration, Other w/ Respiratory Sx	P24.81	
933.1	Foreign Body, Larynx (Choke)	T17.3-±√	
934.9	Foreign Body, Respiratory	T17.9-±√	

ICD-9-CM		ICD-10-CM	
987.1	Gasoline Inhalation	T59.894√	Undetermined
	E869.8 Accidental	T59.891√	
	E952.8 Intentional	T59.892√	
786.39	Hemoptysis, Other Coughing Up Blood	R04.2	
327.22	High-altitude Periodic Breathing	G47.32	
786.01	Hyperventilation	R06.4	
748.5	Hypoplasia, Lung	Q33.6	
799.02	Hypoxia	R09.02	
770.88	Hypoxia, Newborn	P84	
748.3	Laryngomalacia, Tracheomalacia	Q31.5	Laryngomalacia
		Q32.0	Tracheomalacia
861.21	Lung Contusion	S27.322	Bilateral
		S27.321	Unilateral
		S27.329	Unspec
770.12	Meconium Aspiration w/ Respiratory Sx	P24.01	
997.32	Pneumonia, Post-procedural Aspiration	J95.89+	to identify disorder
V12.61	Pneumonia (Recurrent), Hx of	Z87.01	
860.0	Pneumothorax, Traumatic	S27.0XX√	
799.1	Respiratory Arrest	R09.2	
770.87	Respiratory Arrest of Newborn	P28.81	
786.9	*Respiratory Complaints/Sx Breath-holding Spells*	R06.89	
V12.69	Respiratory Disease, Other, Hx of	Z87.09	
V12.60	Respiratory Disease, Unspec, Hx of	Z87.09	
770.84	Respiratory Failure, Newborn	P28.5	
770.89	Respiratory Problems, Newborn, Other	P28.89	
E869.4	Secondhand Smoke Exposure	Z77.22	Secondhand Smoke Exposure
V15.89	Secondhand Smoke Exposure, Hx of		
786.05	Shortness of Breath	R06.02	

8. Diseases of the Respiratory System *(cont)*

ICD-9-CM		ICD-10-CM
DISEASES OF THE RESPIRATORY SYSTEM **Other Related Diagnoses** *(cont)*		
327.23	Sleep Apnea, Obstructive	**G47.33**
327.20	Sleep Apnea, Organic, Unspec	**G47.30**
327.21	Sleep Apnea, Primary Central	**G47.31**
958.7	SQ Emphysema, Traumatic	**T79.7XX√**
786.1	Stridor	**R06.1**
786.06	Tachypnea	**R06.82**
750.3	Tracheoesophageal Fistula	**Q39.1**
997.31	Ventilator-Associated Pneumonia	**J95.851+** *to identify organism*
786.07	Wheezing	**R06.2**

9. Diseases of the Digestive System

ICD-10-CM codes are not valid for use at the time of publication and should not be reported until the official implementation date set by the Centers for Medicare & Medicaid Services.

ICD-9-CM		ICD-10-CM	
565.0	Anal Fissure/Tear	K60.2	
569.43	Anal Sphincter Tear (Healed) (Old) (Nontraumatic)	K62.81+	*associated fecal incontinence R15.-*
528.2	Aphthous Ulcer/Canker Sore	K12.0	
540.1	Appendicitis	K35.3	
540.0	Appendicitis w/ Perforation	K35.2	
575.0	Cholecystitis, Acute	K81.0	
574.20	Cholelithiasis w/o Obstruction	K80.20	
558.3	Colitis/Gastroenteritis, Allergic	K52.2+	*identify type of food allergy Z91.01-, Z91.02-*
556.9	Colitis, Ulcerative, Unspec Site	K51.90	
564.09	Constipation, Other	K59.09	
564.02	Constipation, Outlet Dysfunction	K59.02	
564.01	Constipation, Slow Transit	K59.01	
564.00	Constipation, Unspec	K59.00	
521.81	Cracked Tooth	K03.81	
555.1	Crohn's Disease of Large Intestine	K50.10+	Large Intestine w/o Complications
555.0	Crohn's Disease of Small Intestine	K50.00+	Small Intestine w/o Complications
555.9	*Crohn's Disease, Unspec Site*	K50.90+	Unspec Site, w/o Complications
528.5	Cyst, Lip	K13.0	
522.5	Dental Abscess	K04.7	
521.00	*Dental Caries*	K02.9	
535.60	Duodenitis w/o Hemorrhage	K29.80	
558.42	Eosinophilic Colitis	K52.82	
530.13	Eosinophilic Esophagitis	K20.0	
535.71	Eosinophilic Gastritis, w/ Hemorrhage	K52.81£	
535.70	Eosinophilic Gastritis, w/o Hemorrhage	K52.81£	
558.41	Eosinophilic Gastroenteritis	K52.81£	
526.0	Eruption Cyst (Gum)	K09.0	

9. Diseases of the Digestive System *(cont)*

ICD-9-CM		ICD-10-CM	
530.12	Esophagitis, Acute	K20.9	
560.32	Fecal Impaction	K56.41	
564.9	*Functional Disorder of Intestine*	K59.9	
535.00	Gastritis, Acute w/o Hemorrhage	K29.00	
558.9	Gastroenteritis, Acute, Noninfectious	K52.89	
530.81	Gastroesophageal Reflux	K21.0	w/ Esophagitis
		K21.9	w/o Esophagitis
536.41	Gastrostomy Site Infection	K94.22	
529.1	Geographic Tongue	K14.1	
578.9	*GI Bleeding*	K92.2	
523.8	Gingival Hyperplasia	K06.1	
523.00	Gingivitis, Acute	K05.00	
529.0	Glossitis	K14.0	
578.0	Hematemesis	K92.0	
571.49	Hepatitis, Chronic Nonviral	K73.2	Hepatitis, Chronic, Nonviral, Active
573.1	Hepatitis w/ Infectious Mononucleosis code Mononucleosis (075) first	K77*	*mononucleosis B27.90*
573.5	Hepatopulmonary Syndrome*	K76.81*	*underlying liver disease*
553.3	Hernia, Hiatal	K44.9	
550.90	Hernia, Inguinal	K40.90	
553.1	Hernia, Umbilical	K42.9	
553.20	Hernia, Ventral	K43.3	
560.30	Impaction of Colon	K56.49	
536.8	Indigestion/Dyspepsia	K30	
579.9	*Intestinal Malabsorption*	K90.9	
560.9	*Intestinal Obstruction*	K56.60	
560.0	Intussusception	K56.1	
564.1	Irritable Bowel Syndrome	K58.0	w/ Diarrhea
		K58.9	w/o Diarrhea
524.4	Malocclusion	M26.4	

ICD-9-CM		ICD-10-CM
578.1	Melena/Blood in Stool	K92.1
524.04	Micrognathia	M26.04
579.8	*Milk/Formula Intolerance*	K90.4
520.6	Neonatal Teeth	K00.6
528.3	Oral Cellulitis and Abscess	K12.2
528.9	*Oral Complaints/Sx*	K13.7-
524.29	Overbite	M26.29
577.0	Pancreatitis, Acute	K85.9
560.1	Paralytic Ileus	K56.0
527.2	Parotitis/Sialoadenitis	K11.20
533.90	*Peptic Ulcer w/o Obstruction* add 041.86 if due to Helicobacter pylori	K27.9
566	Perianal Abscess	K61.0
567.21	Peritonitis (Acute), Generalized	K65.0
569.0	Polyp, Rectal	K62.1
521.89	Poor Dentition	K03.89
537.81	Pylorospasm	K31.3
569.42	Rectal/Anal Pain	K62.89
569.3	Rectal Bleeding	K62.5
569.1	Rectal Prolapse	K62.3
555.1	Regional Enteritis of Large Intestine	See Crohn's Disease
555.0	Regional Enteritis of Small Intestine	See Crohn's Disease
555.9	*Regional Enteritis, Unspec Site*	See Crohn's Disease
579.3	Short Gut Syndrome	K91.2
528.00	Stomatitis	K12.1
520.7	Teething Syndrome	K00.7
524.60	TMJ Disorder	M26.60
524.64	TMJ Sounds on Jaw Movement	M26.69

9. Diseases of the Digestive System *(cont)*

ICD-9-CM	ICD-10-CM
525.1Ø Tooth Loss, Acquired	**KØ8.1Ø9** Tooth Loss (Complete), Acquired
	KØ8.4Ø9 Tooth Loss (Partial), Acquired
525.13 Tooth Loss, Caries	**KØ8.139** Tooth Loss (Complete), Caries
	KØ8.439 Tooth Loss (Partial), Caries
525.12 Tooth Loss, Periodontal Disease	**KØ8.129** Tooth Loss (Complete), Periodontal Disease
	KØ8.429 Tooth Loss (Partial), Periodontal Disease
525.11 Tooth Loss, Trauma	**KØ8.119** Tooth Loss (Complete), Trauma
	KØ8.419 Tooth Loss (Partial), Trauma
556.9 Toxic Megacolon	**K51.9Ø**
56Ø.2 Volvulus	**K56.2**
569.87 Vomiting of Fecal Matter	**R11.13**
536.2 Vomiting, Persistent (Nonpregnancy)	**R11.1Ø**

Other Related Diagnoses	
789.9 *Abdominal Complaints/Sx Umbilical Bleeding/Discharge/ Problems*	**R19.8**
787.3 Abdominal Distention/Bloating	**R14.Ø**
789.ØØ Abdominal Pain, Unspec Site	**R1Ø.9**
789.6Ø *Abdominal Tenderness, Unspec Site*	**R1Ø.819**
789.3Ø *Abdominal/Umbilical Mass/ Swelling*	**R19.ØØ**
ØØ6.Ø Amebiasis, Acute	**AØ6.Ø**
863.89 Anal Sphincter Tear, Traumatic	**S36.899√**
783.Ø Anorexia	**R63.Ø**
Ø22.2 Anthrax, GI	**A22.2**
789.51 Ascites, Malignant	**R18.Ø*** *malignancy*
789.59 Ascites, Other	**R18.8**
751.1 Atresia/Stenosis, Small Intestine	**Q41.9**

ICD-9-CM		ICD-10-CM	
751.69	Bile Duct/Gallbladder Anomaly	Q44.5	Bile Duct Anomaly
		Q44.Ø	Gallbladder Agenesis, Aplasia or Hypoplasia
		Q44.1	Gallbladder Anomaly, Other
751.61	Biliary Atresia	Q44.2	Biliary Atresia
		Q44.3	Biliary Stenosis and Stricture
787.Ø4	Bilious Emesis/Vomiting	R11.14	
596.89	Bladder, Distended	N32.89	
V85.51	BMI <5% for Age	Z68.51	
V85.52	BMI 5%–<85% for Age	Z68.52	
V85.53	BMI 85%–<95% for Age	Z68.53	
V85.54	BMI ≥95% for Age	Z68.54	
3Ø7.51	Bulimia	F5Ø.2	
ØØ8.43	Campylobacter Enteritis	AØ4.5	
112.Ø	Candida, Oral (Thrush)	B37.Ø	excludes neonatal
		P37.5	neonatal
112.85	Candidal Enteritis	B37.82	
112.84	Candidal Esophagitis	B37.81	
789.7	Colic, Infantile	R1Ø.83	
751.9	*Congenital Anomaly, GI*	Q45.9	
756.6	Diaphragmatic Hernia	Q79.Ø	
ØØ9.2	Diarrhea/Dysentery, Infectious	AØ9	
787.91	Diarrhea (Noninfectious)	R19.7	
ØØ9.3	Diarrhea, Presumed Infectious	AØ9	
V65.3	Diet Surveillance and Counseling	Z71.3+	*underlying medical condition and BMI if known Z68.-*
787.21	Dysphagia, Oral Phase	R13.11	
787.22	Dysphagia, Oropharyngeal Phase	R13.12	
787.29	Dysphagia, Other	R13.19	
787.23	Dysphagia, Pharyngeal Phase	R13.13	
787.24	Dysphagia, Pharyngoesophageal Phase	R13.14	
787.2Ø	Dysphagia, Unspec	R13.1Ø	

9. Diseases of the Digestive System *(cont)*

ICD-9-CM		ICD-10-CM	
Other Related Diagnoses *(cont)*			
008.00	E. coli Enteritis, Unspec	A04.4	
008.04	E. coli, Enterohemorrhagic	A04.3	
008.01	E. coli, Enteropathogenic	A04.0	
008.02	E. coli, Enterotoxigenic	A04.1	
307.50	Eating Disorder, Atypical	F50.9	
307.7	Encopresis, Nonorganic	F98.1+	*identify cause of any coexisting constipation*
787.60	Fecal Incontinence	R15.9	
787.62	Fecal Soiling	R15.1	
787.63	Fecal Urgency	R15.2	
005.9	Food Poisoning	A05.9	
935.1	Foreign Body, Esophagus	T18.1-±√	
938	Foreign Body, GI	T18.8XX√	
009.0	Gastroenteritis, Infectious	A09	
009.1	Gastroenteritis, Presumed Infectious	N/A	
756.73	Gastroschisis	Q79.3	
V44.1	Gastrostomy Present	Z93.1	
V55.1	Gastrostomy Tube Problem Clogged Dislodged	Z43.1	
787.1	Heartburn	R12	
455.6	Hemorrhoids	K64.-	
455.8	Hemorrhoids, Bleeding	K64.-	
789.1	Hepatomegaly	R16.0	
054.2	Herpetic Gingivostomatitis	B00.2	
751.3	Hirschsprung Disease	Q43.1	
751.2	Imperforate Anus	Q42.9	
V69.1	Inappropriate Diet/Eating Habits	Q43.0	
869.0	*Internal Injury/Blunt Trauma*	S36.90X√	
V45.72	Intestine, Acquired Absence Appendectomy	Z90.49	
873.43	Laceration, Lip	S01.511√	
873.60	Laceration, Mouth	S01.502√	
873.64	Laceration, Tongue	S01.512√	
271.3	Lactase Deficiency	E73.0	Congenital
		E73.1	Secondary

ICD-9-CM		ICD-10-CM
289.2	Lymphadenitis, Mesenteric	I88.0
751.0	Meckel Diverticulum	Q43.0
787.02	Nausea (Alone)	R11.0
787.01	Nausea and Vomiting	R11.2
756.72	Omphalocele	Q79.2
278.02	Overweight	E66.3
	add code for BMI if known	Z68.-
129	Parasitism, Intestinal, Unspec	B82.9
127.4	Pinworms	B80
211.3	Polyposis, Familial	D12.6
V45.89	Postoperative Status excludes transplants, prosthesis placement, removal of kidney and intestine, major organ and heart surgery	Z98.89
698.0	Pruritus Ani	L29.0
750.5	Pyloric Stenosis	Q40.0
008.61	Rotavirus Enteritis	A08.0
865.02	Ruptured Spleen	S36.030√
003.0	Salmonella Gastroenteritis	A02.2
V45.79	Splenectomy Status Post	Z90.89
789.2	Splenomegaly	R16.1
289.53	Splenomegaly, Neutropenic	D73.81
792.1	Stool, Abnormal	R19.5
848.1	Strain, TMJ	S03.4XX√
787.99	Tenesmus (Rectal)	R19.8
750.0	Tongue Tie/Ankyloglossia	Q381
783.22	Underweight	R63.6
	add code for BMI if known	Z68.-
787.03	Vomiting (Alone)	R11.11
787.04	Vomiting, Bilious	R11.14
779.32	Vomiting, Bilious, Newborn	P92.01
779.33	Vomiting, Non-bilious, Newborn	P92.09
783.1	Weight Gain, Abnormal	R63.5
783.21	Weight Loss, Abnormal	R63.4
	add code for BMI if known	Z68.-

10. Diseases of the Genitourinary System

ICD-10-CM codes are not valid for use at the time of publication and should not be reported until the official implementation date set by the Centers for Medicare & Medicaid Services.

ICD-9-CM		ICD-10-CM	
626.0	Amenorrhea	N91.2	
628.0	Anovulatory Cycle	N97.0	
607.1	Balanitis/Balanoposthitis	N48.1+	Balanitis *identify infection B95–B97*
		N47.6+	Balanoposthitis *identify infection B95–B97*
616.3	Bartholin Gland Abscess	N75.1	
616.2	Bartholin Gland Cyst	N75.0	
596.89	Bladder, Distended	N32.89	
596.51	Bladder, Hyperactivity	N32.81	
596.0	Bladder Neck Obstruction	N32.0	
611.72	Breast Lump or Mass	N63	
611.71	Breast Pain	N64.4	
611.79	*Breast Problems*	N64.59	
616.0	Cervicitis	N72+	*identify infection B95–B97*
585.1	Chronic Kidney Disease, Stage 1	N18.1	
585.2	Chronic Kidney Disease, Stage 2 (Mild)	N18.2	
585.3	Chronic Kidney Disease, Stage 3 (Moderate)	N18.3	
585.4	Chronic Kidney Disease, Stage 4 (Severe)	N18.4	
585.5	Chronic Kidney Disease, Stage 5	N18.5	
585.9	Chronic Kidney Disease, Unspec	N18.9	
595.0	Cystitis, Acute	N30.00	Acute Cystitis w/o Hematuria
		N30.01	w/ Hematuria
626.8	Dysfunctional Uterine Bleeding	N93.8	
625.3	Dysmenorrhea	N94.6	
585.6	End-stage Renal Disease	N18.6+	*identify dialysis status Z99.2*
604.90	Epididymitis-Orchitis	N45.1+	Epididymitis *identify infection B95–B97*
		N45.2+	Orchitis *identify infection B95–B97*
625.9	*Female Genital Pain, Nonspecific*	R10.2	

ICD-9-CM		ICD-10-CM	
6Ø5	Foreskin, Adhesion/Excess	N47.5	
611.6	Galactorrhea	N64.3	
58Ø.9	Glomerulonephritis, Acute	NØØ.9	
611.1	Gynecomastia/Hypertrophy (Male or Female)	N62	
599.71	Hematuria, Gross	R31.Ø	
599.72	Hematuria, Microscopic	R31.1	Benign Essential
		R31.2	Other
6Ø3.9	Hydrocele (Not Neonate)	N43.3	
591	Hydronephrosis	N13.3Ø	
623.2	Labial Adhesion	N89.5	
6Ø8.9	*Male Genital Pain*	R1Ø.2	
611.Ø	Mastitis	N61	
598.9	Meatal Stenosis	N35.9	
597.89	Meatitis	N34.2	
626.2	Menstruation, Excessive/Frequent Menorrhagia/Menometrorrhagia	N92.1	w/ Irregular Cycle
		N92.Ø	w/ Regular Cycle
626.4	Menstruation, Irregular Cycle	N92.6	
626.5	Menstruation, Normal Cycle	N92.3	
626.3	Menstruation, Pubertal	N92.2	
626.6	Metrorrhagia/Non-menstrual Bleeding	N92.1	
625.2	Mittelschmerz	N94.Ø	
581.9	Nephrotic Syndrome	NØ4.9	
62Ø.2	Ovarian Cyst	N83.29	Ovarian Cysts, Other (Simple Cysts)
		N83.2Ø	Ovarian Cysts, Unspec
614.9	Pelvic Inflammatory Disease	N73.9	
6Ø7.83	Penis, Edema	N48.89	
6Ø5	Phimosis/Paraphimosis	N47.1	Phimosis
		N47.2	Paraphimosis
625.4	Premenstrual Tension Syndrome	N94.3+	*associated menstrual migraines G43.82-, G43.83-*

10. Diseases of the Genitourinary System *(cont)*

ICD-9-CM		ICD-10-CM	
607.3	Priapism	N48.32*	Due to Disease Classified Elsewhere (Sickle Cell)
		N48.30*	Unspec
601.0	Prostatitis, Acute	N41.0*	*to identify infectious agent B95–B97*
593.6	Proteinuria, Postural	R80.2	
590.10	Pyelonephritis, Acute	N10*	*to identify infectious agent B95–B97*
593.2	Renal Cyst, Acquired	N28.1	
584.9	Renal (Kidney) Failure, Acute	N17.9+	*underlying condition*
592.0	Renal Stone	N20.2	
608.89	Scrotal/Testicular Mass	N44.2	
608.1	Spermatocele	N43.40	
608.3	Testicle, Atrophy	N50.0	
608.9	*Testicular Pain*	N50.89	
608.24	Torsion of Appendix Epididymis	N44.04	
608.23	Torsion of Appendix Testis	N44.03	
608.20	Torsion of Testicle, Unspec	N44.00	
614.2	Tubo-ovarian Abscess	N70.93	
592.1	Ureter Stone	N20.1	
597.80	Urethritis, Non-STD	N34.1	
599.60	Urinary Obstruction, Unspec	N13.9	
599.0	UTI	N39.0+	*to identify infectious agent B95–B97*
623.8	Vaginal Bleeding/Hemorrhage	N89.8	
623.5	Vaginal Discharge, Noninfectious	N89.8	
623.4	Vaginal Tear (Nontraumatic)	N89.8	
593.70	Vesicoureteral Reflux w/o Nephropathy	N13.71	
625.8	Vulvar Mass	N94.89	
616.10	Vulvovaginitis	N76.0+	*to identify infectious agent B95–B97*

ICD-9-CM		ICD-10-CM	
Other Related Diagnoses			
V47.5	Absent Testicle	Q55.0	
759.89	Alport Disease	Q87.81+	*to identify stage of chronic kidney disease N18.1–N18.6*
788.5	Anuria/Oliguria	R34	
772.8	Bleeding, Circumcision, Newborn	P54.8	
112.1	Candidal Vulvovaginitis	B37.3	
995.53	Child Abuse, Sexual/Rape+	T74.22X√	Child Abuse, Sexual Confirmed
		T76.22X√	Child Abuse, Sexual, Suspected
099.55	Chlamydia, GU, Unspec	A56.2	
079.98	Chlamydia, Unspec (Non-STD)	A74.9	
099.41	Chlamydia Urethritis (STD)	A56.01	
752.63	Chordee, Congenital	Q54.4	
752.9	*Congenital Anomaly, Genital*	Q52.9	Female
		Q55.9	Male
753.9	*Congenital Anomaly, Urinary*	Q64.9	
753.10	Cystic Kidney Disease	Q61.9	
259.0	Delayed Puberty	E30.0	
788.1	Dysuria	R30.0	
788.36	Enuresis, Nocturnal	N39.44	
307.6	Enuresis, Nonorganic	F98.0	
752.62	Epispadias	Q64.0	
V01.6	Exposure to STD	Z20.2	
753.5	Exstrophy of Bladder	Q64.10	
939.2	Foreign Body, Vagina	T19.2XX√	
098.15	Gonococcal Cervicitis	A54.03	
098.17	Gonococcal Salpingitis	A54.24	
098.0	Gonorrhea, Acute	A54.00	
	Gonococcal Urethritis	A54.01	
	Gonococcal Vulvovaginitis	A54.02	
791.2	Hemoglobinuria (Microscopic)	R82.3	
550.90	Hernia, Inguinal	K40.90	
054.10	Herpes, Genital	A60.00	

10. Diseases of the Genitourinary System *(cont)*

ICD-9-CM		ICD-10-CM
Other Related Diagnoses *(cont)*		
778.6	Hydrocele, Congenital/Newborn	P83.5
753.29	Hydronephrosis, Congenital	Q62.0
752.61	Hypospadias	Q54.9
752.42	Imperforate Hymen	Q52.3
752.7	Indeterminate Sex	Q56.4
V45.73	Kidney, Acquired Absence	Z90.5
752.49	Labial Adhesion, Congenital	Q52.8
878.8	Laceration, External/Genitalia	S31.512√ Female
		S31.511√ Male
V13.03	Nephrotic Syndrome, Hx of	Z87.441
194.0	Neuroblastoma	C74.90∞
V71.5	Obs for Alleged (Child) Rape Exam for Alleged (Child) Rape	Z04.42
132.2	Pediculosis, Genital	B85.3
752.69	Penile Anomalies	Q55.69
752.65	Penis, Hidden	Q55.64
752.64	Penis, Micro	Q55.62
753.12	Polycystic Kidney	Q61.3
256.4	Polycystic Ovaries	E28.2
788.42	Polyuria	R38.5
259.1	Precocious Sexual Development	E30.1
V72.41	Pregnancy Test, Negative	Z32.02
V72.42	Pregnancy Test, Positive	Z32.01
V72.40	Pregnancy Test, Pregnancy Unconfirmed	Z32.00
791.0	Proteinuria	R80.9
698.1	Pruritus, Genital Organs	L29.1 Scroti
		L29.3 Unspec
		L29.2 Vulvae
788.0	Renal Colic	N23
866.00	Renal Contusion	S37.009√
753.11	Renal Cyst, Congenital	Q61.01
753.15	Renal Dysplasia	Q61.4

ICD-9-CM		ICD-10-CM	
V42.Ø	Renal Transplant Present	Z94.Ø	
453.3	Renal Vein Thrombosis	I82.3	
V67.59	STD, Follow-up Exam	ZØ9	
Ø99.9	*STD, Unspec*	A64	
Ø91.Ø	Syphilis, Genital (Primary)	A51.Ø	
752.52	Testis, Retractile	Q55.22	
752.51	Testis, Undescended	Q53.9	
11Ø.3	Tinea cruris (Groin)	B35.6	
959.14	Trauma, GU/Pelvis/Perineum	S39.848√	GU/Perineum
		S39.83X√	Pelvis
131.Ø9	Trichomonal Cervicitis	A59.Ø9	
131.Ø2	Trichomonal Urethritis	A59.Ø3	
131.Ø1	Trichomonal Vulvovaginitis	A59.Ø1	
753.23	Ureterocele, Congenital	Q62.31	
753.21	Ureteropelvic Obstruction, Congenital	Q62.11	
753.22	Ureterovesical Obstruction, Congenital	Q62.12	
788.7	Urethral Discharge	R36.9	
Ø99.4Ø	Urethritis, Nonspecific (STD)	N34.1	
788.9	*Urinary Complaints/Sx*	R39.89	
V13.ØØ	Urinary Disorders, Unspec, Hx of	Z87.448	
788.41	Urinary Frequency	R35.Ø	
788.64	Urinary Hesitancy	R39.11	
788.3Ø	Urinary Incontinence	R32	
788.63	Urinary Urgency	R39.15	
878.6	Vaginal Tear/Laceration (Traumatic)	S31.4ØX√	
456.4	Varicocele	I86.1	
Ø78.11	Warts, Genital	A63.Ø	
189.Ø	Wilms Tumor	C64.2	Left Kidney
		C64.1	Right Kidney
		C64.9	Unspec Kidney

11. Complications of Pregnancy, Childbirth, and the Puerperium

ICD-10-CM codes are not valid for use at the time of publication and should not be reported until the official implementation date set by the Centers for Medicare & Medicaid Services.

ICD-9-CM		ICD-10-CM
632	Abortion, Missed	O02.1
634.90	Abortion, Spontaneous	O03.9
640.03	Abortion, Threatened	O20.0
633.1	Pregnancy, Ectopic (Tubal)	O00.1
659.80	Pregnancy, <16 Years of Age at Delivery	O75.89

Other Related Diagnoses		
V25.03	Contraception, Emergency Counseling and Prescription	Z30.012
V25.02	Contraception Initiation, IUD	Z30.014
V25.01	Contraception Initiation, Oral	Z30.011
V25.40	*Contraception Surveillance*	Z30.40
V25.42	Contraceptive Monitoring, IUD includes removal and reinsertion	Z30.430 Encounter for Insertion of IUD
		Z30.432 Encounter for Removal of IUD
		Z30.433 Encounter for Removal and Reinsertion of IUD
		Z30.431 Routine Checking of IUD
V25.41	Contraceptive Monitoring, Oral includes repeat prescription	Z30.41
762.5	Cord Around Neck at Delivery	P02.5
V25.09	Family Planning Advice	Z30.09
V23.84	High-risk Pregnancy, Young Multigravida <16 Years of Age at Expected Delivery	O09.62±
V23.83	High-risk Pregnancy, Young Primigravida <16 Years of Age at Expected Delivery	O09.61±
		±For High-risk Pregnancy Codes, Use 6th Digit 1 = First Trimester; 2 = Second Trimester; 3 = Third Trimester; 9 = Unspec Trimester

ICD-9-CM		ICD-10-CM
V25.04	*Natural Family Planning Counseling to Avoid Pregnancy*	Z30.02
V26.49	Pregnancy Counseling	Z31.69
V72.41	Pregnancy Test, Negative	Z32.02
V72.42	Pregnancy Test, Positive	Z32.01
V72.40	Pregnancy Test, Pregnancy Unconfirmed	Z32.00
V22.2	Pregnant	Z33.1
V89.03	Suspected Fetal Anomaly Not Found	Z03.73
V89.04	Suspected Problem w/ Fetal Growth Not Found	Z03.74
762.6	Umbilical Cord Hematoma	P02.69

12. Diseases of the Skin and Subcutaneous Tissue

ICD-10-CM codes are not valid for use at the time of publication and should not be reported until the official implementation date set by the Centers for Medicare & Medicaid Services.

ICD-9-CM		ICD-10-CM	
682.9	*Abscess/Lymphangitis, Unspec*	L03.91	
701.2	Acanthosis Nigricans	L83	
706.1	Acne	L70.4	Acne, Infantile
		L70.9	Acne, Unspec
		L70.0	Acne Vulgaris
704.00	Alopecia/Hair Loss	L65.9	
691.8	Atopic Dermatitis/Eczema	L20.89	
680.9	*Boil/Carbuncle/Furuncle, Unspec*	L02.93	Carbuncle, Unspec
		L02.92	Furuncle, Unspec (Boil)
709.09	Café au Lait Spots	L81.3	
682.9	*Cellulitis, Unspec*	L03.90	
700	Corns/Callus	L84	
690.18	Dandruff	L21.8	
707.00	*Decubitus Ulcer, Unspec Site*	L89.90	
709.3	Degenerative Skin Disorders	L98.8	
	Calcification/Deposits, SQ/Skin	L94.2	
	SQ Fat Necrosis	L98.8	
692.9	*Dermatitis, Contact, Unspec*	L23.9	
692.84	Dermatitis, Due to Animal Hair/Dander	L23.81	
692.4	Dermatitis, Due to Chemical	L23.5	
692.81	Dermatitis, Due to Cosmetics	L23.2	
693.9	Dermatitis, Due to Ingested Substances	L27.2	
692.83	Dermatitis, Due to Metal/Jewelry	L23.0	
692.6	Dermatitis, Due to Plants/Poison Ivy, Oak	L23.7	
692.82	Dermatitis, Due to Tanning Equipment	L56.8 and W89.1XX√	
698.4	Dermatitis Factitia	L98.1	
691.0	Diaper Rash	L22	
709.00	Dyschromia, Skin	L81.8	
	Hyperpigmentation	L81.4	
	Hypopigmentation	L81.8	
705.81	Dyshidrosis	L30.1	

ICD-9-CM		ICD-10-CM	
695.12	Erythema Multiforme Major	L51.8	
695.11	Erythema Multiforme Minor	L51.8	
695.2	Erythema Nodosum	L52	
681.01	Felon	L03.019	
704.8	Folliculitis/Ingrown Hair	L73.8	
709.4	Granuloma, Foreign Body	L92.3	
686.1	Granuloma, Pyogenic Umbilical Cord Granuloma	L98.0	
705.1	Heat Rash/ Miliaria Rubra	L74.0	
	Sudamina	L74.1	
705.83	Hidradenitis	L73.2	
704.1	Hirsutism	L68.0	
684	Impetigo	L01.00	
703.0	Ingrown Nail	L60.0	
695.89	Intertrigo	L30.4	
701.4	Keloid Scar	L91.0	
683	Lymphadenitis, Acute	L04.9	
703.8	Nail Abnormalities/Diseases	L60.8	
	Onycholysis	L60.1	
681.02	Paronychia/Onychia, Finger	L03.01±	
681.11	Paronychia/Onychia, Toe	L03.02±	
		±For Paronychia Codes, Use 6th Digit 1 = Right Side; 2 = Left Side; 9 = Unspec	
692.79	Photosensitivity (Solar)	L56.8	
704.41	Pilar Cyst	L72.11	
685.1	Pilonidal Sinus/Cyst w/o Abscess	L05.91	Cyst
		L05.91	Sinus
696.3	Pityriasis Rosea	L42	
698.0	Pruritus Ani	L29.0	
698.1	Pruritus, Genital Organs	L29.1	Scroti
		L29.3	Unspec
		L29.2	Vulvae
698.9	*Pruritus/Itch*	L29.9	

12. Diseases of the Skin and Subcutaneous Tissue *(cont)*

ICD-9-CM		ICD-10-CM	
686.Ø1	Pyoderma, Gangrenosum	L88	
686.ØØ	Pyoderma, Unspec	LØ8.Ø	
695.81	Ritter Disease	LØØ	
7Ø9.2	Scar/Disfigurement	L9Ø.5	
7Ø6.2	Sebaceous (Skin) Cyst	L72.3	
7Ø6.3	Seborrhea	L21.9	
69Ø.11	Seborrhea Capitis (Cradle Cap)	L21.Ø	
69Ø.1Ø	Seborrheic Dermatitis	L21.8	
69Ø.12	Seborrheic Infantile Dermatitis	L21.1	
686.9	Skin Infection, Unspec	LØ8.9	
7Ø1.9	Skin Tag, Acquired	L91.9	
695.13	Stevens-Johnson Syndrome	L51.1	
695.14	Stevens-Johnson Syndrome–Toxic Epidermal Necrolysis Overlap Syndrome	L51.3*+	*to identify associated manifestations to identify percentage of skin exfoliation L49.-*
692.71	Sunburn, First Degree	L55.Ø	
692.76	Sunburn, Second Degree	L55.1	
692.77	Sunburn, Third Degree	L55.2	
695.15	Toxic Epidermal Necrolysis	L51.2	
7Ø4.42	Trichilemmal Cyst	L72.12	
7Ø8.Ø	Urticaria, Allergic	L5Ø.Ø	
7Ø8.8	Urticaria, Chronic/Recurrent	L5Ø.8	
7Ø8.9	Urticaria/Hives, Unspec	L5Ø.9	
7Ø9.Ø1	Vitiligo	L8Ø	

Other Related Diagnoses			
443.89	Acrocyanosis	I73.89	
995.2Ø	Adverse Effect, Medication, Unspec	T5Ø.9Ø5√	
287.Ø	Allergic Purpura (Schönlein-Henoch)	D69.Ø	
995.3	Allergic Reaction, Non-medication	T78.3XX√	
995.1	Angioneurotic Edema	T78.4ØX√	

ICD-9-CM		ICD-10-CM	
307.9	Behavior Activities Nail Biting Thumb Sucking	F98.8	
949.1	Burn, First Degree, Unspec Site	T30.0XX√	not for inpatient use
941.00	Burn, Head/Face/Neck, Unspec Degree	T20.00X+√	*external cause code to* *identify source, place,* *and intent of burn*
945.00	Burn, Lower Limb, Unspec Degree	T24.009+√	*external cause code to* *identify source, place,* *and intent of burn*
949.2	*Burn, Second Degree,* *Unspec Site*	T30.0XX√	not for inpatient use
949.3	*Burn, Third Degree, Unspec Site*	T30.0XX√	not for inpatient use
942.00	Burn, Trunk, Unspec Degree	T21.00X√+	*external cause code to* *identify source, place,* *and intent of burn*
949.0	*Burn, Unspec Site/Degree*	T30.0XX√	not for inpatient use
943.00	Burn, Upper Limb, Unspec Degree	T22.00X+√	*external cause code to* *identify source, place,* *and intent of burn*
944.00	Burn, Wrist, Hand, Unspec Degree	T23.009+√	*external cause code to* *identify source, place,* *and intent of burn*
112.3	Candidiasis of Skin and Nails	B37.2	
757.9	*Congenital Anomaly, Integument*	Q84.9	
757.39	*Congenital Anomaly, Skin* *(Specific)*	Q82.8	
	Cutis Aplasia		
	Epidermolysis Bullosa	Q81.-	
	Skin Tags, Congenital		
757.32	*Congenital Vascular Hamartomas* Birthmark Port-wine Stain Strawberry Nevus	Q82.5	

12. Diseases of the Skin and Subcutaneous Tissue (cont)

ICD-9-CM		ICD-10-CM	
Other Related Diagnoses (cont)			
924.9	*Contusion*	T14.8	
922.31	Contusion, Back	S30.0XX√	
922.32	Contusion, Buttock	S30.0XX√	
922.33	Contusion, Interscapular	S20.229√	
929.0	*Crush Injury*	T07.-√	
772.6	Cutaneous Hemorrhage, Newborn	P54.5	
710.3	Dermatomyositis	M33.90	
110.9	Dermatophytosis, Ringworm	B39.5	
995.27	Drug Allergy/Hypersensitivity	T50.995√	
782.3	Edema/Swelling	R60.9	
756.83	Ehlers-Danlos Syndrome	Q79.6	
035	Erysipelas	A46	
778.8	Erythema Toxicum, Newborn	P83.1	
919.7	*Foreign Body, Skin w/ Infection*	T07.-√	
919.6	*Foreign Body, Skin w/o Infection*	T07.-√	
228.01	Hemangioma, Skin	D18.01	
228.00	*Hemangioma, Unspec Site Cavernous Hemangioma*	D18.00	
053.9	Herpes Zoster	B02.9	
780.8	Hyperhidrosis/Excessive Sweating	R61	
919.5	*Insect Bite w/ Infection, Unspec Site*	T07.-√	
919.4	*Insect Bite w/o Infection, Unspec Site*	T07.-√	
880.02	Laceration/Bite/Puncture, Axillae	S41.019√	Laceration, Axillae, Unspec Side
		S41.059√	Bite, Open, Axillae, Unspec Side
		S41.039√	Puncture, Axillae, Unspec Side
873.40	*Laceration/Bite/Puncture, Face*	S01.91X√	Laceration Unspec Part of Head
		S01.95X√	Bite, Open, Unspec Part of Head
		S01.93X√	Puncture, Unspec Part of Head

ICD-9-CM		ICD-10-CM	
883.Ø	Laceration/Bite/Puncture, Finger(s)	S61.219√	Laceration, Unspec Finger, w/o Nail Damage
		S61.259√	Bite, Open, Unspec Finger, w/o Nail Damage
		S61.239√	Puncture, Unspec Finger, w/o Nail Damage
892.Ø	Laceration/Bite/Puncture, Foot	S91.319√	Laceration, Unspec Foot
		S91.359√	Bite, Open, Unspec Foot
		S91.339√	Puncture, Unspec Foot
882.Ø	Laceration/Bite/Puncture, Hand	S61.419√	Laceration, Unspec Hand
		S61.459√	Bite, Open, Unspec Hand
		S61.439√	Puncture, Unspec Hand
894.Ø	Laceration/Bite/Puncture, Lower Extremity	S81.819√	Laceration, Unspec Lower Leg
		S81.859√	Bite, Open, Unspec Lower Leg
		S81.839√	Puncture, Unspec, Lower Leg
874.8	Laceration/Bite/Puncture, Neck	S11.91X√	Laceration Unspec Part of Neck
		S11.95X√	Bite, Open, Unspec Part of Neck
		S11.93X√	Puncture, Unspec Part of Neck
873.Ø	Laceration/Bite/Puncture, Scalp	SØ1.Ø1X√	Laceration, Scalp
		SØ1.Ø5X√	Bite, Open, Scalp
		SØ1.Ø3X√	Puncture, Scalp
893.Ø	Laceration/Bite/Puncture, Toe(s)	S91.119√	Laceration, Unspec Toe, w/o Nail Damage
		S91.159√	Bite, Open, Unspec Toe, w/o Nail Damage
		S91.139√	Puncture, Unspec Toe, w/o Nail Damage

12. Diseases of the Skin and Subcutaneous Tissue *(cont)*

ICD-9-CM		ICD-10-CM	
Other Related Diagnoses *(cont)*			
879.6	Laceration/Bite/Puncture, Trunk	S31.010√	Laceration, Trunk
		S31.050√	Bite, Open, Trunk
		S31.030√	Puncture, Trunk
884.0	Laceration/Bite/Puncture, Upper Extremity	S41.119√	Laceration, Unspec Upper Extremity
		S41.159√	Bite, Open, Unspec Upper Extremity
		S41.139√	Puncture, Unspec Upper Extremity
214.1	Lipoma Skin/SQ	D17.-	
088.81	Lyme Disease	A69.2-	
785.6	Lymphadenopathy	R59.1	
078.0	Molluscum Contagiosum	B08.1	
237.70	Neurofibromatosis, Unspec	Q85.00	
216.9	Nevus, Unspec Site Pigmented, Skin, Giant, Hairy, Mole(s)	D23.9	
782.61	Pallor	R23.1	
132.1	Pediculosis, Body	B85.1	
132.0	Pediculosis, Head	B85.0	
782.7	Petechiae	R23.3	
696.1	Psoriasis	L40.8	
287.2	Purpura	D69.2	
782.1	*Rash*	R21	
133.0	Scabies	B86	
782.2	*Skin Mass/Lump/Nodule*	R22.-	
778.1	SQ Fat Necrosis, Newborn	P83.0	
927.3	Subungual Hematoma of Finger	S67.10X√	Finger, Unspec
		S67.00X√	Thumb, Unspec
928.3	Subungual Hematoma of Toe	S97.119√	Great Toe, Unspec
		S97.109√	Toes, Unspec
919.8	*Superficial Injury, Unspec w/o Infection*	T07.-√	
757.6	Supernumerary Nipple	Q83.3	

ICD-9-CM		ICD-10-CM	
120.3	Swimmer's Itch	B65.3	
710.0	Systemic Lupus Erythematosus+	M32.10	
110.0	Tinea capitis (Scalp)	B35.0	
110.5	Tinea corporis (Body)	B35.4	
110.3	Tinea cruris (Groin)	B35.6	
110.4	Tinea pedis (Feet)	B35.3	
111.0	Tinea versicolor	B36.0	
989.5	Venomous Bite	T63.91X√	Venomous Bite, Unspec Animal, Accidental
	Bee	T63.441√	Accidental
	Jellyfish	T63.621√	Accidental
	Snake	T63.001√	Snake, Unspec, Accidental
	Spider	T63.301√	Spider, Unspec, Accidental
	Tick	T63.481√	Accidental
057.9	Viral Exanthem	B09	Viral Exanthem, NOS
078.19	Warts, Common	B07.8	
078.12	Warts, Plantar	B07.0	
272.2	Xanthoma	E78.2	

13. Diseases of the Musculoskeletal System and Connective Tissue

ICD-10-CM codes are not valid for use at the time of publication and should not be reported until the official implementation date set by the Centers for Medicare & Medicaid Services.

ICD-9-CM		ICD-10-CM	
726.71	Achilles Tendinitis	M76.60	Unspec Leg
727.81	Achilles Tendon Contracture	M67.00	Unspec Ankle
733.91	Arrested Bone Growth Delayed Bone Age	M89.1-	
716.90	*Arthritis, Unspec*	M12.9	
716.10	*Arthropathy, Traumatic*	M12.50	
713.8	Arthropathy, w/ Associated Condition*	M14.80*	
727.51	Baker Cyst	M71.20	Unspec Knee
733.20	Bone Cyst	M85.60	
736.42	Bowlegs/Genu Varum, Acquired	M21.169	Unspec
727.1	Bunion	M20.10	Unspec Foot
727.3	Bursitis	M71.50	
717.7	Chondromalacia Patellae	M22.40	Unspec Knee
724.79	Coccygodynia	M53.3	
733.6	Costochondritis/Tietze Disease	M94.0	
738.10	Deformity, Head, Acquired	M95.2	
710.3	Dermatomyositis+	M33.90	
719.7	Difficulty Walking/Limp	R26.2	
719.07	Effusion/Swelling, Ankle	M25.473	Unspec Ankle
719.02	Effusion/Swelling, Elbow	M25.429	Unspec Elbow
719.06	Effusion/Swelling, Knee	M25.469	Unspec Knee
719.03	Effusion/Swelling, Wrist	M25.439	Unspec Wrist
710.5	Eosinophilia Myalgia Syndrome+§	M35.8	
726.91	Exostosis/Bone Spur	M25.70	Unspec Joint
729.4	Fasciitis	M72.9	
728.86	Fasciitis, Necrotizing	M72.6+	*to identify causative organism B95.-, B96.-*
727.43	Ganglion	M67.40	Unspec Site
719.10	Hemarthrosis, Nontraumatic	M25.00	
714.30	Juvenile Rheumatoid Arthritis	M08.00+	Unspec Site
736.41	Knock-knee/Genu Valgum	M21.069	

ICD-9-CM		ICD-10-CM	
732.1	Legg-Calvé-Perthes Disease	M91.8Ø	Unspec Leg
728.81	Limb Swelling	M6Ø.1Ø	Unspec Site
737.2Ø	Lordosis	M4Ø.4Ø	Unspec Site
724.2	Lumbago/Low Back Pain	M54.5	
729.82	Muscle Cramps	R25.2	
728.85	Muscle Spasm	M62.838	
728.87	Muscle Weakness	M62.81	
729.1	Myalgia/Myositis	M79.1	Myalgia
		M6Ø.9	Myostitis, Unspec
728.Ø	Myositis, Infective	M6Ø.ØØ9	Myositis, Infective, Unspec Site
732.4	Osgood-Schlatter Disease	M92.52	Left Leg
		M92.51	Right Leg
		M92.5Ø	Unspec Leg
732.9	Osteochondrosis, Unspec	M92.9	
73Ø.ØØ	*Osteomyelitis, Acute, Unspec* add 731.3 w/ major osseous defect	M86.1Ø+	*to identify infectious agent B95–B97 if applicable, report M89.7- to identify major osseous defect*
731.Ø	Paget Disease	M88.-	
719.47	Pain, Ankle	M25.579∞	
724.5	Pain, Back	M54.9	
719.42	Pain, Elbow	M25.529∞	
719.45	Pain, Hip	M25.559∞	
719.46	Pain, Knee	M25.569∞	
729.5	Pain, Limb Non-joint Pain in Extremity, Hand, Foot	M79.6Ø3∞	Pain in Arm, Unspec
		M79.6Ø6∞	Pain in Leg, Unspec
		M79.6Ø9	Pain in Unspec Limb
719.43	Pain, Wrist	M25.539∞	
73Ø.3Ø	Periostitis	M86.9	
734	Pes Planus/Flatfeet, Acquired	M21.4Ø∞	
711.ØØ	*Pyogenic Arthritis*	MØØ.9	

13. Diseases of the Musculoskeletal System and Connective Tissue *(cont)*

ICD-9-CM		ICD-10-CM	
728.88	Rhabdomyolysis	M62.82	
727.61	Rotator Cuff, Complete Tear	M75.120∞	
726.13	Rotator Cuff, Partial Tear	M75.110∞	
737.30	Scoliosis	M41.129	Scoliosis, Adolescent, Idiopathic, Unspec Site
		M41.00	Scoliosis, Infantile Idiopathic, Unspec Site
		M41.119	Scoliosis, Juvenile Idiopathic, Unspec Site
732.5	Sever Disease/Calcaneal Epiphysitis	M92.60∞	
732.2	Slipped Capital Femoral Epiphysis	M93.003∞	
723.1	Sore Neck	M54.2	
719.57	Stiffness, Ankle	M25.673∞	
719.52	Stiffness, Elbow	M25.629∞	
719.56	Stiffness, Knee	M25.669∞	
719.53	Stiffness, Wrist	M25.639∞	
733.94	Stress Fx, Metatarsals	M84.375√	Left Foot
		M84.374√	Right Foot
		M84.376√	Unspec Foot
733.95	Stress Fx, Other Bone	M84.38X√	
733.93	Stress Fx, Tibia or Fibula	M84.362√	Left Tibia
		M84.361√	Right Tibia
		M84.364√	Left Fibula
		M84.363√	Right Fibula
		M84.369√	Unspec Tibia or Fibula
710.0	Systemic Lupus Erythematosus+	M32.10	
727.00	Tenosynovitis	M65.9	
736.89	Tibial Torsion	M21.969∞	
723.5	Torticollis/Wry Neck	M43.6	

ICD-9-CM		ICD-10-CM	
Other Related Diagnoses			
755.55	Acrocephalosyndactyly Apert Syndrome	Q87.0	
755.63	Anteversion of Femur	Q65.89	
754.89	Arthrogryposis Multiplex Congenita	Q74.3	
995.54	Battered Child Syndrome	T74.12X¤	Child Neglect, Confirmed
		T76.12X¤	Child Neglect, Suspected
343.9	Cerebral Palsy, Infantile, Unspec	G80.9	
754.70	*Clubfoot, Congenital*	Q66.89	
755.60	*Congenital Anomaly, Lower Extremity*	Q74.2	
756.9	*Congenital Anomaly, Musculoskeletal*	Q79.9	
755.50	*Congenital Anomaly, Upper Extremity*	Q74.9	
754.70	*Congenital Deformity, Feet*	Q66.89	
759.89	*Congenital Malformation Syndromes*	Q89.8+	*to identify all associated manifestations*
	Alport Syndrome	Q87.81+	*to identify stage of chronic kidney disease N18.1–N18.6*
	Beckwith-Wiedemann Syndrome	Q87.3	
	Hemihypertrophy	Q89.8+	*to identify all associated manifestations*
	Noonan Syndrome	Q87.1	
927.3	Crushed Finger(s)	S67.10X√	Finger, Unspec
		S67.00X√	Thumb, Unspec
834.00	Dislocation, Finger, Closed	S36.259√	Finger, Unspec
		S36.106√∞	Thumb
754.30	Dislocation, Hip, Unilateral, Congenital	Q65.00∞	
836.50	Dislocation, Knee, Closed	S83.105√	Dislocation, Knee, Left
		S83.104√	Dislocation, Knee, Right
		S83.106√	Dislocation, Knee, Unspec

13. Diseases of the Musculoskeletal System and Connective Tissue *(cont)*

ICD-9-CM		ICD-10-CM	
Other Related Diagnoses *(cont)*			
836.3	Dislocation/Subluxation, Patella, Closed	S83.005√	Dislocation, Patella, Left
		S83.004√	Dislocation, Patella, Right
		S83.006√	Dislocation, Patella, Unspec
		S83.003√∞	Subluxation, Patella, Unspec
259.4	Dwarfism, Endocrine	E34.3	
755.63	Dysplasia, Hip, Congenital	Q65.89	
754.51	Equinovarus, Congenital	Q66.0	
170.7	Ewing Sarcoma, Lower Limb	C40.2-	
170.4	Ewing Sarcoma, Upper Limb	C40.0-	
824.8	Fx Ankle, Unspec, Closed	S82.899√	
805.00	Fx Cervical, Closed	S12.9XX√	
810.00	Fx Clavicle, Closed	S42.009√∞	
767.2	Fx Clavicle, Newborn	P13.4	
821.00	Fx Femur, Closed	S72.90X√∞	
823.41	Fx Fibula, Torus/Buckle	S82.829√∞	Lower End
		S82.819√∞	Upper End
816.00	Fx Finger(s)/Phalange(s) (Hand), Closed	S62.609√	Finger, Unspec
		S62.509√∞	Thumb
825.20	Fx Foot/Metatarsal, Closed	S92.909√∞	
813.80	Fx Forearm, Unspec, Closed	S52.90X√∞	
815.00	Fx Hand/Metacarpal, Closed	S62.309√∞	
812.20	Fx Humerus, Closed	S42.309√∞	
802.20	Fx Mandible, Closed	S02.609√+	*associated intracranial injury S06.-*
808.8	Fx Pelvis, Unspec, Closed	S32.9XX√	
813.45	Fx Radius, Torus/Buckle	S52.119√∞	

ICD-9-CM		ICD-10-CM	
813.47	Fx Radius/Ulna, Torus/Buckle	S52.129√∞ Radius, Lower End, Torus	
		S52.119√∞ Radius, Upper End, Torus	
		S52.629√∞ Ulna, Lower End, Torus	
		S52.009√∞ Ulna, Upper End, Torus	
807.00	Fx Rib(s), Closed	S22.39X√∞	
823.40	Fx Tibia, Torus/Buckle	See S82.319 and S82.169 Below	
823.82	Fx Tibia/Fibula, Closed	S82.209√∞ Tibia	
		S82.409√∞ Fibula	
823.42	Fx Tibia/Fibula, Torus/Buckle	S82.319√∞ Tibia, Lower End, Torus	
		S82.169√∞ Tibia, Upper End, Torus	
		S82.829√∞ Fibula, Lower End, Torus	
		S82.819√∞ Fibula, Upper End, Torus	
826.0	Fx Toe(s)/Phalange(s) (Foot), Closed	S92.406√	Great Toe, Unspec
		S92.506√	Lesser Toe(s), Unspec
813.46	Fx Ulna, Torus/Buckle	See S52.- Above	
814.00	Fx Wrist/Carpal, Closed	S92.109√∞	
781.2	Gait Abnormality	R26.0	Gait Abnormalities, Staggering
		R26.2	Difficulty in Walking, NEC
		R26.1	Spastic Gait
781.99	*Growing Pains*	R29.91	
342.90	Hemiplegia	G81.92	Unspec, Affecting Left Dominant Side
		G81.94	Unspec, Affecting Left Nondominant Side
		G81.91	Unspec, Affecting Right Dominant Side
		G81.93	Unspec, Affecting Right Nondominant Side
		G81.90	Unspec, Affecting Unspec Side

13. Diseases of the Musculoskeletal System and Connective Tissue *(cont)*

ICD-9-CM		ICD-10-CM	
Other Related Diagnoses *(cont)*			
342.00	Hemiplegia, Flaccid	**G81.02**	Flaccid Hemiplegia Affecting Left Dominant Side
		G81.04	Flaccid Hemiplegia Affecting Left Nondominant Side
		G81.01	Flaccid Hemiplegia Affecting Right Dominant Side
		G81.03	Flaccid Hemiplegia Affecting Right Nondominant Side
		G81.00	Flaccid Hemiplegia Affecting Unspec Side
342.10	Hemiplegia, Spastic	**G81.12**	Spastic Hemiplegia Affecting Left Dominant Side
		G81.14	Spastic Hemiplegia Affecting Left Nondominant Side
		G81.11	Spastic Hemiplegia Affecting Right Dominant Side
		G81.13	Spastic Hemiplegia Affecting Right Nondominant Side
		G81.10	Spastic Hemiplegia Affecting Unspec Side
844.9	Injury, Knee Ligament	S83.90X√∞	
840.4	Injury, Rotator Cuff	S43.429√∞	
V13.4	Juvenile Rheumatoid Arthritis, Hx of	Z87.39	
759.82	Marfan Syndrome	Q87.40	
754.53	Metatarsus Varus/Adductus	Q66.2	
524.04	Micrognathia	M26.04	

ICD-9-CM		ICD-10-CM	
277.5	Mucopolysaccharide Disease	E76.3	Mucopolysaccharide Disease, Unspec
	Hunter Syndrome	E76.1	
	Hurler Syndrome	E76.Ø1	
	Morquio-Brailsford Disease	E76.21Ø	Morquio A Mucopolysaccharidoses
		E76.211	Morquio B Mucopolysaccharidoses
		E76.219	Morquio Mucopolysaccharidoses, Unspec
359.1	Muscular Dystrophy, Hereditary	G71.Ø	
781.99	*Musculoskeletal Complaints/Sx*	R29.91	
358.9	*Neuromuscular Disorder*	G7Ø.9	
832.2	Nursemaid Elbow	S53.Ø33√∞	
V71.89	Obs for Juvenile Rheumatoid Arthritis	ZØ3.89	
756.51	Osteogenesis Imperfecta	Q78.Ø	
784.92	Pain, Jaw	R68.84	
344.1	Paraplegia	G82.21	Paraplegia, Complete
		G82.22	Paraplegia, Incomplete
		G82.2Ø	Paraplegia, Unspec
754.82	Pectus Carinatum/Pigeon Chest, Congenital	Q67.7	
754.81	Pectus Excavatum, Congenital	Q67.6	
754.61	Pes Planus/Rocker Bottom Foot, Congenital	Q66.5Ø∞	
755.Ø1	Polydactyly/Accessory Fingers	Q69.Ø	Finger(s)
		Q69.1	Thumb
755.Ø2	Polydactyly/Accessory Toes	Q69.2	
344.ØØ	Quadriplegia	G82.5Ø	
755.2Ø	Short Arm Length, Congenital	Q71.813	Bilateral
		Q71.819∞	Unspec Arm
755.3Ø	Short Leg Length, Congenital	Q72.813	Bilateral
		Q72.819∞	Unspec Leg
756.12	Spondylolisthesis, Congenital	Q76.2	

13. Diseases of the Musculoskeletal System and Connective Tissue *(cont)*

ICD-9-CM		ICD-10-CM
Other Related Diagnoses *(cont)*		
845.00	Sprain/Strain, Ankle	S93.409√∞
841.9	Sprain/Strain, Elbow	S53.409√∞
845.10	Sprain/Strain, Foot/Toe	S93.609√∞ Foot
		S93.503√∞ Great Toe
		S93.506√∞ Other Unspec Toe
842.10	Sprain/Strain, Hand/Finger	S63.90X√∞ Hand
		S63.619√∞ Other Unspec Finger
		S63.609√∞ Thumb
844.9	Sprain/Strain, Knee	S83.90X√∞
846.0	Sprain/Strain, Lumbosacral	S33.8XX√
847.0	Sprain/Strain, Neck/Whiplash	S13.4XX√
842.00	Sprain/Strain, Wrist	S63.509√∞
754.32	Subluxation/Click, Hip, Congenital	Q65.30∞ Subluxation, Hip
		R29.4 Hip Click
755.10	*Syndactyly*	Q70.9 Syndactyly, Unspec
524.60	TMJ Disorder	M26.60
524.64	TMJ Sounds on Jaw Movement	M26.69
754.1	Torticollis, Congenital	Q68.0
781.93	Torticollis, Ocular	R29.891
335.0	Werdnig-Hoffmann Disease	G12.0

14. Congenital Anomalies

ICD-10-CM codes are not valid for use at the time of publication and should not be reported until the official implementation date set by the Centers for Medicare & Medicaid Services.

ICD-9-CM		ICD-10-CM	
757.6	Absence of Breast or Nipple	Q83.Ø	
755.55	Acrocephalosyndactyly Apert Syndrome	Q87.Ø	
742.2	Agenesis Corpus Callosum	QØ4.Ø	
756.Ø	Anomalies Skull/Face Megalocephaly/Large Head Premature Closure of the Sutures	Q75.8	
755.63	Anteversion of Femur	Q65.89	
746.3	Aortic Stenosis	Q23.Ø	
754.89	Arthrogryposis Multiplex Congenita	Q74.3	
751.1	Atresia/Stenosis, Small Intestine	Q41.9	
745.5	Atrial Septal Defect	Q21.1	
745.69	Atrioventricular Canal	Q21.2	
758.39	Autosomal Deletion Syndrome, Other	Q93.89	
751.69	Bile Duct/Gallbladder Anomaly	Q44.5	Bile Duct Anomaly
		Q44.Ø	Gallbladder Agenesis, Aplasia or Hypoplasia
		Q44.1	Gallbladder Anomaly, Other
751.61	Biliary Atresia	Q44.2	Biliary Atresia
		Q44.3	Biliary Stenosis and Stricture
743.3Ø	Cataract, Congenital, Unspec	Q12.Ø	
752.63	Chordee, Congenital	Q54.4	
758.9	Chromosome Anomalies, Unspec	Q99.9	
749.1Ø	*Cleft Lip*	Q36.Ø	Bilateral
		Q36.1	Median
		Q36.9	Unilateral (NOS)
749.ØØ	*Cleft Palate*	Q35.1	Cleft Hard Palate
		Q35.5	Cleft Hard Palate w/Cleft Soft Palate
		Q35.9	Cleft Palate, Unspec
		Q35.3	Cleft Soft Palate

14. **Congenital Anomalies** *(cont)*

ICD-9-CM		ICD-10-CM	
754.7Ø	*Clubfoot, Congenital*	**Q66.89**	
747.1Ø	Coarctation of Aorta	**Q25.1**	
743.46	Coloboma Iris	**Q13.Ø**	
759.7	*Congenital Anomalies, Multiple*	**Q89.7**	
742.9	*Congenital Anomaly, CNS*	**QØ7.9**	
744.3	*Congenital Anomaly, Ear*	**Q17.9**	
743.9	*Congenital Anomaly, Eye*	**Q15.9**	
744.9	*Congenital Anomaly, Face/Neck*	**Q18.9**	
752.9	*Congenital Anomaly, Genital*	**Q52.9**	Female
		Q55.9	Male
751.9	*Congenital Anomaly, GI*	**Q45.9**	
757.9	*Congenital Anomaly, Integument*	**Q84.9**	
755.6Ø	*Congenital Anomaly, Lower Extremity*	**Q74.2**	
756.9	*Congenital Anomaly, Musculoskeletal*	**Q79.9**	
748.9	*Congenital Anomaly, Respiratory*	**Q34.9**	
757.39	*Congenital Anomaly, Skin (Specific)* **Cutis Aplasia** **Epidermolysis Bullosa**	**Q82.8**	
755.5Ø	*Congenital Anomaly, Upper Extremity*	**Q74.9**	
753.9	*Congenital Anomaly, Urinary*	**Q64.9**	
754.7Ø	*Congenital Deformity, Feet*	**Q66.89**	
754.Ø	*Congenital Deformity, Skull/Face*	**Q67.4**	
746.9	*Congenital Heart Disease, Unspec*	**Q24.9**	
759.89	*Congenital Malformation Syndromes*	**Q89.8+**	*to identify all associated manifestations*
	Alport Syndrome	**Q87.81+**	*to identify stage of chronic kidney disease N18.1–N18.6*
	Beckwith-Wiedemann Syndrome	**Q87.3**	
	Hemihypertrophy	**Q89.8+**	*to identify all associated manifestations*
	Noonan Syndrome	**Q87.1**	

ICD-9-CM		ICD-10-CM	
757.32	*Congenital Vascular Hamartomas* Birthmark Port-wine Stain Strawberry Nevus	Q82.5	
758.31	Cri Du Chat Syndrome	Q93.4	
753.10	Cystic Kidney Disease	Q61.9	
756.6	Diaphragmatic Hernia	Q79.0	
754.30	Dislocation, Hip, Unilateral, Congenital	Q65.00∞	
755.63	Dysplasia, Hip, Congenital	Q65.89	
756.83	Ehlers-Danlos Syndrome	Q79.6	
745.60	Endocardial Cushion Defect	Q21.2	
752.62	Epispadias	Q64.0	
753.5	Exstrophy of Bladder	Q64.10	
747.83	Fetal Circulation, Persistent	P29.3	
759.83	Fragile X Syndrome	Q99.2	
756.73	Gastroschisis	Q79.3	
743.20	Glaucoma, Congenital	Q15.0	
751.3	Hirschsprung Disease	Q43.1	
742.3	Hydrocephalus, Congenital	Q03.0	Malformations of Aqueduct of Sylvius
	Dandy-Walker Cyst	Q03.1	
		Q03.8	Other
		Q03.9	Unspec
753.29	Hydronephrosis, Congenital	Q62.0	
748.5	Hypoplasia, Lung	Q33.6	
746.7	Hypoplastic Left Heart	Q23.4	
752.61	Hypospadias	Q54.9	
751.2	Imperforate Anus	Q42.9	
758.7	Klinefelter (XXY) Syndrome	Q98.4	
752.49	Labial Adhesion, Congenital	Q52.8	
748.3	Laryngomalacia, Tracheomalacia	Q31.5	Laryngomalacia
		Q32.0	Tracheomalacia
759.82	Marfan Syndrome	Q87.40	

14. Congenital Anomalies *(cont)*

ICD-9-CM		ICD-10-CM	
751.0	Meckel Diverticulum	Q43.0	
754.53	Metatarsus Varus/Adductus	Q66.2	
742.1	Microcephalus, Congenital	Q02	
758.33	Microdeletions (Autosomal), Other Miller-Dieker Syndrome Smith-Magenis Syndrome	Q93.88	
741.93	Myelomeningocele, Lumbar	Q05.7	
748.0	Nasal Stenosis/Choanal Atresia	Q30.0	
756.72	Omphalocele	Q79.2	
756.51	Osteogenesis Imperfecta	Q78.0	
747.0	Patent Ductus Arteriosus	Q25.0	
754.82	Pectus Carinatum/Pigeon Chest, Congenital	Q67.7	
754.81	Pectus Excavatum, Congenital	Q67.6	
752.69	Penile Anomalies	Q55.69	
752.65	Penis, Hidden	Q55.64	
752.64	Penis, Micro	Q55.62	
754.61	Pes Planus/Rocker Bottom Foot, Congenital	Q66.50∞	
753.12	Polycystic Kidney	Q61.3	
755.01	Polydactyly/Accessory Fingers	Q69.0	Finger(s)
		Q69.1	Thumb
755.02	Polydactyly/Accessory Toes	Q69.2	
742.4	Porencephalic Cyst	Q04.6	excludes acquired
759.81	Prader-Willi Syndrome	Q87.1	
756.71	Prune Belly Syndrome	Q79.4	
743.61	Ptosis, Congenital	Q10.0	
747.32	Pulmonary Arteriovenous Malformation	Q25.72	
747.39	Pulmonary Artery Anomalies	Q25.79	
747.31	Pulmonary Artery Coarctation and Atresia Hypoplasia Stenosis	Q25.5	
746.02	Pulmonary Valve Stenosis	Q22.1	

ICD-9-CM		ICD-10-CM	
750.5	Pyloric Stenosis	Q40.0	
753.11	Renal Cyst, Congenital	Q61.01	
753.15	Renal Dysplasia	Q61.4	
758.81	Sex Chromosome Anomalies, Other	Q97.9	Female Phenotype
		Q98.9	Male Phenotype
	XXX Female Syndrome	Q97.0	
	XYY Syndrome	Q98.5	
755.20	Short Arm Length, Congenital	Q71.813	Bilateral
		Q71.819∞	Unspec Arm
755.30	Short Leg Length, Congenital	Q72.813	Bilateral
		Q72.819∞	Unspec Leg
747.5	Single Umbilical Artery	Q27.0	
759.3	Situs Inversus Kartagener Syndrome	Q89.3	
741.00	Spina Bifida w/ Hydrocephalus	Q05.4	
	Arnold-Chiari Syndrome Type II	Q07.03	
741.90	Spina Bifida w/o Hydrocephalus	Q05.8	
756.12	Spondylolisthesis, Congenital	Q76.2	
757.32	*Strawberry Nevus/Birthmark*	Q82.5	
759.6	Sturge-Weber Syndrome	Q85.8	
754.32	Subluxation/Click, Hip, Congenital	Q65.30∞	Subluxation, Hip
		R29.4	Hip Click
757.6	Supernumerary Nipple	Q83.3	
755.10	*Syndactyly*	Q70.9	Syndactyly, Unspec
752.52	Testis, Retractile	Q55.22	
752.51	Testis, Undescended	Q53.9	
745.2	Tetralogy of Fallot	Q21.3	
759.2	Thyroglossal Duct Cyst	Q89.2	
750.0	Tongue Tie/Ankyloglossia	Q381	
754.1	Torticollis, Congenital	Q68.0	
747.41	Total Anomalous Pulmonary Venous Return	Q26.2	
750.3	Tracheoesophageal Fistula	Q39.1	
745.10	Transposition of Great Vessels	Q20.3	

14. Congenital Anomalies *(cont)*

ICD-9-CM		ICD-10-CM	
758.1	Trisomy 13/Patau Syndrome	Q91.4	Patau Syndrome
		Q91.7	Trisomy 13, Unspec
758.2	Trisomy 18/Edward Syndrome	Q91.Ø	Edward Syndrome
		Q91.3	Trisomy 18, Unspec
758.Ø	Trisomy 21/Down Syndrome	Q9Ø.9	
745.Ø	Truncus Arteriosus	Q2Ø.Ø	
758.6	Turner (XO) Syndrome	Q96.9	
753.23	Ureterocele, Congenital	Q62.31	
753.21	Ureteropelvic Obstruction, Congenital	Q62.11	
753.22	Ureterovesical Obstruction, Congenital	Q62.12	
758.32	Velocardiofacial Syndrome	Q93.81	
745.4	Ventricular Septal Defect	Q21.Ø	

Other Related Diagnoses			
V13.67	Congenital Malformations of Digestive System, Hx of (Corrected)	Z87.738	
V13.64	Congenital Malformations of Eye, Ear, Face, and Neck, Hx of (Corrected)	Z87.73Ø	Cleft Lip/Palate
		Z87.721	Ear
		Z87.72Ø	Eye
		Z87.79Ø	Face/Neck
V13.65	Congenital Malformations of Heart and Circulatory System, Hx of (Corrected)	Z87.74	
V13.68	Congenital Malformations of Integument, Limbs, and Musculoskeletal System, Hx of (Corrected)	Z87.76	
V13.63	Congenital Malformations of Nervous System, Hx of (Corrected)	Z87.728	
V13.62	Congenital Malformations of Other GU System, Hx of (Corrected)	Z87.718	

ICD-9-CM		ICD-10-CM
V13.66	Congenital Malformations of Respiratory System, Hx of (Corrected)	Z87.75
V13.69	Congenital Malformations, Other, Hx of (Corrected)	Z87.798
243	Hypothyroidism, Congenital	E03.1
352.6	Möbius Syndrome	G52.7
796.6	Neonatal Screen, Nonspecific Abnormal Finding	P09
V29.3	Obs for Genetic or Metabolic Condition, Newborn	P00.89
779.89	Other Perinatal Condition	P96.89+ *to specify condition*
	Congenital Hypotonia	P94.2
362.75	Retinal Cone Dystrophy	H35.53

15. Certain Conditions Originating in the Perinatal Period (<29 Days Of Age)

ICD-10-CM codes are not valid for use at the time of publication and should not be reported until the official implementation date set by the Centers for Medicare & Medicaid Services.

ICD-9-CM		ICD-10-CM	
773.1	ABO Hemolytic Disease, Newborn	P55.1	
762.1	Abruptio Placentae, Affecting Infant	P02.1	
775.81	Acidosis, Newborn	P84	
776.6	Anemia of Prematurity	P61.2	
770.82	Apnea, Newborn, Other	R28.4	
770.81	Apnea, Primary of Newborn	R28.3	
771.83	Bacteremia, Newborn	R78.81	Bacteremia
768.6	Birth Asphyxia, Mild/Moderate w/o CNS Sx	P84	
768.5	Birth Asphyxia, Severe w/ CNS Sx	P84	
768.9	Birth Asphyxia, Unspec	P84	
767.8	Birth Trauma, Other Injured Viscus	P15.8	
	Eye Damage	P15.3	
	Scalp Wound	P12.9	
766.0	Birth Weight ≥4,500 g	P08.0	
772.8	Bleeding, Circumcision, Newborn	P54.8	
772.3	Bleeding, Umbilicus, Newborn	P51.8	
767.6	Brachial Plexus Injury, Newborn	P14.3	
	Erb Palsy	P14.0	
	Klumpke Palsy	P14.1	
779.81	Bradycardia, Newborn	P29.12	
778.7	Breast Engorgement, Newborn	P83.4	
770.7	Bronchopulmonary Dysplasia	P27.1	
771.7	Candidal Infection of Newborn Monilia Thrush	P37.5	
779.85	Cardiac Arrest of Newborn	P29.81	
767.19	Cephalohematoma, Newborn	P12.0	
767.0	Cerebral Hemorrhage, Newborn	P10.1	
762.7	Chorioamnionitis, Affecting Infant	P02.7	

ICD-9-CM		ICD-10-CM	
779.2	CNS Dysfunction, Newborn	P91.4	Cerebral Depression, Neonatal
		P91.0	Cerebral Ischemia, Neonatal
		P91.5	Coma, Neonatal
		P91.9	Unspec
771.6	Conjunctivitis/Dacryocystitis, Newborn	P39.1	
779.0	Convulsions, Newborn	P90	
762.5	Cord Around Neck at Delivery	P02.5	
770.83	Cyanosis, Newborn	P28.2	
771.1	Cytomegalovirus Infection, Congenital	P35.1	
779.83	Delayed Umbilical Cord Separation	P96.82	
763.0	Delivery, Breech, Affecting Infant	P03.0	
763.4	Delivery, Cesarean, Affecting Infant	P03.4	
763.2	Delivery, Forceps, Affecting Infant	P03.2	
763.89	Delivery, Other Condition, Affecting Infant	P03.89	
763.3	Delivery, Vacuum, Affecting Infant	P03.3	
775.1	Diabetes Mellitus, Neonatal	P70.2	
776.2	DIC, Newborn	P60	
779.5	Drug Withdrawal Syndrome, Newborn	P96.1	Addicted Drugs
		P96.2	Therapeutic Drugs
778.8	Erythema Toxicum, Newborn	P83.1	
765.01	Extreme Prematurity, <500 g	P07.01	
765.02	Extreme Prematurity, 500–749 g	P07.02	
765.03	Extreme Prematurity, 750–999 g	P07.03	
765.00	Extreme Prematurity, Unspec Weight	P07.00	

15. Certain Conditions Originating in the Perinatal Period (<29 Days Of Age) *(cont)*

ICD-9-CM		ICD-10-CM	
767.5	Facial Nerve Injury/Palsy, Newborn	P11.3	
779.34	Failure to Thrive in Newborn	P92.6	
779.31	Feeding Problems, Newborn	P92.8	
760.71	Fetal Alcohol Syndrome	Q86.0	
770.16	Fetal and Newborn Aspiration of Blood w/ Respiratory Sx	P24.21	
770.15	Fetal and Newborn Aspiration of Blood w/o Respiratory Sx	P24.20	
770.14	Fetal and Newborn Aspiration of Clear Amniotic Fluid w/ Respiratory Sx	P24.11	
770.13	Fetal and Newborn Aspiration of Clear Amniotic Fluid w/o Respiratory Sx	P24.10	
770.86	Fetal and Newborn Aspiration of Postnatal Stomach Contents w/ Respiratory Sx	P24.31	
770.85	Fetal and Newborn Aspiration of Postnatal Stomach Contents w/o Respiratory Sx	P24.30	
770.18	Fetal and Newborn Aspiration, Other w/ Respiratory Sx	P24.81	
770.17	Fetal and Newborn Aspiration, Other w/o Respiratory Sx	P24.80	
770.10	Fetal and Newborn Aspiration, Unspec	P24.9	
772.0	Fetal Blood Loss	P50.9	Unspec
768.3	Fetal Distress Noted During Labor and Delivery	P19.0	Noted Before Onset of Labor
		P19.2	Noted at Birth
		P19.1	Noted During Labor
768.4	Fetal Distress, Unspec Time of Onset	P19.9	
763.83	*Fetal Heart Rate/Rhythm Abnormality*	P03.810	Onset Before Labor
		P03.811	Onset During Labor
		P03.819	Unspec Time of Onset

ICD-9-CM		ICD-10-CM	
778.4	Fever, Newborn	P81.9	Fever, Newborn, NOS
775.5	Fluid and Electrolyte Disturbances, Newborn	P74.4	
767.2	Fx Clavicle, Newborn	P13.4	
767.3	Fx Skull, Newborn/Molded Head	P13.0	
765.21	Gestation, <24 Completed Weeks	P07.21	Gestation <23 Weeks
		P07.22	Gestation 23 Weeks
765.22	Gestation, 24 Completed Weeks	P07.23	Gestation 24 Weeks
765.23	Gestation, 25–26 Completed Weeks	P07.24	Gestation 25 Weeks
		P07.25	Gestation 26 Weeks
765.24	Gestation, 27–28 Completed Weeks	P07.26	Gestation 27 Weeks
		P08.31	Gestation 28 Weeks
765.25	Gestation, 29–30 Completed Weeks	P08.32	Gestation 29 Weeks
		P08.33	Gestation 30 Weeks
765.26	Gestation, 31–32 Completed Weeks	P08.34	Gestation 31 Weeks
		P08.35	Gestation 32 Weeks
765.27	Gestation, 33–34 Completed Weeks	P08.36	Gestation 33 Weeks
		P08.37	Gestation 34 Weeks
765.28	Gestation, 35–36 Completed Weeks	P08.38	Gestation 35 Weeks
		P08.39	Gestation 36 Weeks
765.29	Gestation, ≥37 Completed Weeks	N/A	
766.21	Gestation, Post-term, 40–42 Weeks	P08.21	
766.22	Gestation, Prolonged, >42 Weeks	P08.22	
765.20	Gestation, Unspec Number of Weeks	P07.20	Extreme Immaturity
		P07.30	Preterm
776.0	Hemorrhagic Disease of Newborn Vitamin K Deficiency of Newborn	P53	
774.4	Hepatitis, Neonatal	P59.29	Hepatitis, Neonatal (Jaundice), Due to Other Hepatocellular Damage (Giant Cell Hepatitis)
		P59.20	Hepatitis, Neonatal (Jaundice), Due to Unspec Hepatocellular Damage
		P59.1	Inspissated Bile Syndrome

15. Certain Conditions Originating in the Perinatal Period (<29 Days Of Age) *(cont)*

ICD-9-CM		ICD-10-CM	
778.6	Hydrocele, Congenital/Newborn	P83.5	
775.5	Hypermagnesemia, Newborn	P71.8	
775.4	Hypocalcemia, Newborn	P71.Ø	Cow's Milk Hypocalcemia
		P71.1	Other
775.6	Hypoglycemia, Newborn	P7Ø.4	
778.3	Hypothermia, Newborn	P8Ø.8	Mild
		P8Ø.9	Unspec
77Ø.88	Hypoxia, Newborn	P84	
768.71	Hypoxic-ischemic Encephalopathy, Mild	P91.61	
768.72	Hypoxic-ischemic Encephalopathy, Moderate	P91.62	
768.73	Hypoxic-ischemic Encephalopathy, Severe	P91.63	
768.7Ø	Hypoxic-ischemic Encephalopathy, Unspec	P91.6Ø	
761.Ø	Incompetent Cervix, Affecting Infant	PØ1.Ø	
775.Ø	Infant of Diabetic Mother	PØ7.1	Infant of Diabetic Mother
		PØ7.Ø	Infant of Gestational Diabetic Mother
76Ø.7Ø	Infant of Substance-abusing Mother	PØ4.9	
771.2	Infection, Congenital, Other (Specific)	P37.8	
	Herpes	P35.2	
	Toxoplasmosis	P37.1	
	Listeriosis	P37.2	
771.89	Infection, Other, During Perinatal Period	P39.8	
764.9Ø	Intrauterine Growth Retardation	PØ5.9	
772.11	Intraventricular Hemorrhage, Grade I	P52.Ø	
772.12	Intraventricular Hemorrhage, Grade II	P52.1	
772.13	Intraventricular Hemorrhage, Grade III	P52.21	

ICD-9-CM		ICD-10-CM	
772.14	Intraventricular Hemorrhage, Grade IV	P52.22	
772.10	Intraventricular Hemorrhage, Unspec	P52.3	
774.39	Jaundice, Newborn, Breast Milk	P59.3	
774.6	Jaundice, Newborn, Physiologic Jaundice	P59.9	
774.2	Jaundice of Prematurity	P59.0	
766.1	Large for Gestational Age	P08.1	
761.7	Malpresentation, Affecting Infant	P01.7	
771.5	Mastitis, Infective, Newborn	P39.0	
763.5	Maternal Anesthesia, Affecting Infant	P04.0	
760.2	Maternal Infection, Affecting Infant	P00.2	
760.71	Maternal Use of Alcohol, Affecting Infant	P04.3	
760.77	Maternal Use of Anticonvulsants, Affecting Infant	P04.1	
760.74	Maternal Use of Anti-infectives, Affecting Infant	P04.1	
760.78	Maternal Use of Antimetabolic Agents, Affecting Infant	P04.1	
760.75	Maternal Use of Cocaine, Affecting Infant	P04.41	
760.73	Maternal Use of Hallucinogens, Affecting Infant	P04.49	
760.72	Maternal Use of Narcotics, Affecting Infant	P04.49	
760.79	Maternal Use of Other Medicinals or Toxic Substances, Affecting Infant	P04.1	Medicinal
	Tobacco Use	P04.2	
		P04.8	Toxic Substances
760.70	Maternal Use of Unspec Noxious Substances, Affecting Infant	P04.9	
770.12	Meconium Aspiration w/ Respiratory Sx	P24.01	

15. Certain Conditions Originating in the Perinatal Period (<29 Days Of Age) *(cont)*

ICD-9-CM		ICD-10-CM	
770.11	Meconium Aspiration w/o Respiratory Sx	P24.00	
777.1	Meconium Ileus/Plug	P76.0	
763.84	Meconium Passage During Delivery	P03.82	
779.84	Meconium Staining	P96.83	
777.51	Necrotizing Enterocolitis, Stage 1	P77.1	
777.52	Necrotizing Enterocolitis, Stage 2	P77.2	
777.53	Necrotizing Enterocolitis, Stage 3	P77.3	
777.50	Necrotizing Enterocolitis, Unspec	P77.9	
760.61	Newborn Affected by Amniocentesis	P00.6	
760.62	Newborn Affected by Other In Utero Procedure	P00.7	
760.63	Newborn Affected by Other Surgical Operations on Mother During Pregnancy	P00.7	
760.64	Newborn Affected by Previous Surgical Procedure on Mother Not Associated w/ Pregnancy	P00.6	
771.4	Omphalitis, Newborn	P38.9	
779.89	Other Perinatal Condition	P96.89+	*to specify condition*
	Congenital Hypotonia	P94.2	
779.7	Periventricular Leukomalacia	P91.2	
762.0	Placenta Previa, Affecting Infant	P02.0	
762.2	Placental Insufficiency, Affecting Infant	P02.29	
762.3	Placental Transfusion, Affecting Infant	P02.3	
770.0	Pneumonia, Congenital	P23.-	use specific code to identify infection
770.2	Pneumothorax/ Pneumomediastinum, Newborn	P25.1	Pneumothorax, Neonate
		P25.2	Pneumomediastinum, Neonate
776.4	Polycythemia Neonatorum	P61.1	

ICD-9-CM		ICD-10-CM	
761.1	Premature Rupture of Membranes	P01.1	
765.14	Prematurity, 1,000–1,249 g	P07.14	
765.15	Prematurity, 1,250–1,499 g	P07.15	
765.16	Prematurity, 1,500–1,749 g	P07.16	
765.17	Prematurity, 1,750–1,999 g	P07.17	
765.18	Prematurity, 2,000–2,499 g	P07.18	
765.10	Prematurity, Unspec Weight	P07.10	
770.4	Primary Atelectasis, Newborn	P28.0	
762.4	Prolapsed Cord, Affecting Infant	P02.4	
770.3	Pulmonary Hemorrhage, Newborn	P26.8	
770.87	Respiratory Arrest of Newborn	P28.81	
769	Respiratory Distress Syndrome Hyaline Membrane Disease	P22.0	
770.84	Respiratory Failure, Newborn	P28.5	
770.89	Respiratory Problems, Newborn, Other	P28.89	
	Respiratory Depression	P28.9	
773.0	Rh Hemolytic Disease, Newborn	P55.0	
771.0	Rubella, Congenital	P35.0	
771.81	Sepsis, Newborn	P36.0-	
763.1	Shoulder Dystocia, Affecting Infant	P03.1	
764.0X	Small for Gestational Age	P05.0-	Light for Gestational Age
		P05.1-	Small for Gestational Age
778.1	SQ Fat Necrosis, Newborn	P83.0	
767.11	Subgaleal Hemorrhage	P12.2	
777.3	Swallowed Maternal Blood	P78.2	
779.82	Tachycardia, Newborn	P29.11	
770.6	Transitory Tachypnea of Newborn	P22.1	
762.6	Umbilical Cord Hematoma	P02.69	
771.82	UTI, Newborn	P39.3	
779.32	Vomiting, Bilious, Newborn	P92.01	
779.33	Vomiting, Non-bilious, Newborn	P92.09	

15. Certain Conditions Originating in the Perinatal Period (<29 Days Of Age) *(cont)*

ICD-9-CM		ICD-10-CM	
Other Related Diagnoses			
799.82	ALTE in Newborn or Infant	R68.13*+	*code first a confirmed diagnosis of cause; if there is no confirmed diagnosis, report ALTE (R68.13) in addition to associated signs and Sx*
333.1	Benign Myoclonus of Infancy	G25.3	
277.01	Cystic Fibrosis w/ Meconium Ileus	E84.11	
747.83	Fetal Circulation, Persistent	P29.3	
098.40	Gonococcal Newborn Conjunctivitis	A54.31	
282.43	Hydrops Fetalis Due to Alpha Thalassemia	D56.0	
273.8	Hypoalbuminemia	E88.09	
244.8	Hypothyroidism of Prematurity	E01.8	Iodine Deficiency
		E03.8	Other
V21.31	LBW, <500 g	P07.01	
V21.32	LBW, 500–999 g	P07.02	Extremely LBW Newborn, 500-749 g
		P07.03	Extremely LBW Newborn, 750-999 g
V21.33	LBW, 1,000–1,499 g	P07.1-	See Prematurity
V21.34	LBW, 1,500–1,999 g	P07.1-	See Prematurity
V21.35	LBW, 2,000–2,500 g	P07.1-	See Prematurity
V37.01	Liveborn, Multiple, by Cesarean	Z38.64	Quadruplet
		Z38.62	Triplet
V37.00	Liveborn, Multiple, in Hospital	Z38.63	Quadruplet
		Z38.62	Triplet
V30.01	Liveborn, Single, by Cesarean	Z38.01	
V30.00	Liveborn, Single, in Hospital	Z38.00	
V30.1	Liveborn, Single, Out of Hospital	Z38.1	
V31.01	Liveborn, Twins, by Cesarean	Z38.31	
V31.00	Liveborn, Twins, in Hospital	Z38.30	
V31.1	Liveborn, Twins, Out of Hospital	Z38.4	

ICD-9-CM		ICD-10-CM	
289.7	Methemoglobinemia	D74.8	Methemoglobinemia, Acquired (Toxic)
		D74.Ø	Methemoglobinemia, Congenital
		D74.9	Methemoglobinemia, Unspec
796.6	Neonatal Screen, Nonspecific Abnormal Finding	PØ9	
V29.1	Obs for Neurologic Condition, Newborn Evaluation for Neonatal Seizures	PØØ.89	
V29.8	Obs for Other Suspected Condition, Newborn	PØØ.89	
V29.2	Obs for Respiratory Condition, Newborn Evaluation for Neonatal Apnea	PØØ.3	
V29.Ø	Obs for Suspected Infection, Newborn Evaluation for Sepsis/Infection	PØØ.2	
519.4	Paralysis of Diaphragm	J98.6	
V13.7	Perinatal Problems, Hx of excludes LBW	Z87.898	
786.31	Pulmonary Hemorrhage, Acute Idiopathic in Infants >28 Days	RØ4.81	
695.81	Ritter Disease	LØØ	
747.5	Single Umbilical Artery	Q27.Ø	
Ø41.Ø2	Streptococcus, Group B*	B95.1	
798.Ø	Sudden Infant Death Syndrome	R99	
Ø9Ø.2	Syphilis, Congenital	A5Ø.2	

16. Symptoms, Signs, and Ill-defined Conditions

ICD-10-CM codes are not valid for use at the time of publication and should not be reported until the official implementation date set by the Centers for Medicare & Medicaid Services.

ICD-9-CM		ICD-10-CM	
789.9	*Abdominal Complaints/Sx*	R19.8	
787.3	Abdominal Distention/Bloating	R14.0	
789.00	*Abdominal Pain, Unspec Site*	R10.9	
789.60	*Abdominal Tenderness, Unspec Site*	R10.819	
789.30	*Abdominal/Umbilical Mass/ Swelling*	R19.00	
786.7	Abnormal Chest Sounds (Not Wheezing) Rales Rhonchi	R09.89	
790.3	Alcohol Blood Level Elevated	R78.0+	*for detail regarding alcohol level Y90.-*
799.82	ALTE in Newborn or Infant	R68.13*+	*confirmed diagnosis, use additional code for associated signs and Sx in absence of a confirmed diagnosis*
780.97	Altered Mental Status	R41.82	
783.0	Anorexia	R63.0	
795.31	Anthrax, Nonspecific Positive Findings	R89.9	
788.5	Anuria/Oliguria	R34	
786.03	Apnea	R06.81	
790.91	Arterial Blood Gas, Abnormal	R79.81	
789.51	Ascites, Malignant	R18.0*	*malignancy*
789.59	Ascites, Other	R18.8	
799.01	Asphyxia	R09.01	
781.3	Ataxia	R27.0	
799.51	Attention or Concentration Deficit (Not Associated w/ ADD)	R41.840	
790.7	Bacteremia identify agent w/ appropriate 041 code	R78.81	
787.04	Bilious Emesis	R11.14	
785.9	*Cardiovascular Complaints/Sx*	R09.89	
786.50	Chest Pain	R07.9	

ICD-9-CM		ICD-10-CM
786.04	Cheyne-Stokes Respiration	R06.3
780.64	Chills w/o Fever	R68.83
780.71	Chronic Fatigue Syndrome	R53.82
790.92	Coagulation Profile, Abnormal	R79.1
789.7	Colic, Infantile	R10.83
780.01	Coma	R40.20 Coma, Unspec
786.2	Cough	R05
790.95	C-reactive Protein, Nonspecific Elevation	R79.82
782.5	Cyanosis	R23.0
783.42	Delay in Developmental Milestones	R62.0
783.40	Developmental Delay	R62.50
787.91	Diarrhea (Noninfectious)	R19.7
799.9	Disease, Unknown/Diagnosis Deferred	R69
784.51	Dysarthria	R47.1
784.61	Dyslexia	R48.0
787.21	Dysphagia, Oral Phase	R13.11
787.22	Dysphagia, Oropharyngeal Phase	R13.12
787.29	Dysphagia, Other	R13.19
787.23	Dysphagia, Pharyngeal Phase	R13.13
787.24	Dysphagia, Pharyngoesophageal Phase	R13.14
787.20	Dysphagia, Unspec	R13.10
788.1	Dysuria	R30.0
782.3	Edema/Swelling	R60.9
796.2	*Elevated BP, w/o Hypertension*	R03.0
790.21	Elevated Fasting Glucose	R73.01
788.36	Enuresis, Nocturnal	N39.44
784.7	Epistaxis/Nosebleed	R04.0
780.95	Excessive Crying, Child, Adolescent, or Adult	R45.83
780.92	Excessive Crying, Infant (Baby)	R68.11
783.41	Failure to Thrive	R62.51

16. Symptoms, Signs, and Ill-defined Conditions (cont)

ICD-9-CM		ICD-10-CM	
787.60	Fecal Incontinence	R15.9	
787.62	Fecal Soiling	R15.1	
787.63	Fecal Urgency	R15.2	
783.3	Feeding Problem	R63.3	
780.62	Fever, Post-procedural	R50.82	
780.66	Fever, Posttransfusion FNHTR	R50.84	
780.63	Fever, Postvaccination	R50.83	
780.61	Fever Presenting w/ (Chronic) Conditions Classified Elsewhere*	R50.81*	
780.60	Fever (w/ or w/o Chills)	R50.9	
784.52	Fluency Disorder w/ Conditions Classified Elsewhere*	R47.82*	
780.91	Fussy Infant (Baby)	R68.12	
781.2	Gait Abnormality	R26.0	Gait Abnormalities, Staggering
		R26.2	Difficulty in Walking, NEC
		R26.89	Other
		R26.1	Spastic Gait
		R26.81	Unsteadiness on Feet
791.5	Glycosuria	R81	
781.99	Growing Pains	R29.91	
780.1	Hallucinations	R44.0	Auditory
		R44.3	Unspec
		R44.1	Visual
784.0	Headache	R51	
787.1	Heartburn	R12	
791.2	Hemoglobinuria (Microscopic)	R82.3	
786.39	Hemoptysis, Other Coughing Up Blood	R04.2	
789.1	Hepatomegaly	R16.0	
795.71	HIV Test, Nonspecific Results	R75	
784.42	Hoarseness	R49.0	
790.29	Hyperglycemia	R73.9	
780.8	Hyperhidrosis/Excessive Sweating	R61	

ICD-9-CM		ICD-10-CM	
786.01	Hyperventilation	R06.4	
780.65	Hypothermia Not Associated w/ Low Environmental Temperature	R68.0	
799.02	Hypoxia	R09.02	
790.22	Impaired Oral Glucose Tolerance Test	R73.02	
799.23	Impulsiveness	R45.87	
799.22	Irritability	R45.4	
782.4	Jaundice, Unspec, Not Newborn	R17	
790.6	Lead Test, Positive, Nonspecific	R78.71	
785.6	Lymphadenopathy	R59.1	
780.79	Malaise and Fatigue	R53.83	Fatigue
		R53.81	Malaise
781.6	Meningismus/Stiff Neck	R29.1	
785.2	Murmur, Functional	R01.0	Murmur, Benign and Innocent (Functional)
		R01.1	Murmur, Heart NOS
781.99	*Musculoskeletal/Neurologic Complaints/Sx*	R29.91	Musculoskeletal Complaints/Sx
		R29.90	Neurologic Complaints/Sx
787.02	Nausea (Alone)	R11.0	
787.01	Nausea and Vomiting	R11.2	
796.6	Neonatal Screen, Nonspecific Abnormal Finding	P09	
799.21	Nervousness	R45.0	
783.9	*Other Sx Concerning Nutrition, Metabolism, and Development*	R63. 8	Other Sx Food or Fluid Intake
784.92	Pain, Jaw	R68.84	
782.61	Pallor	R23.1	
785.1	Palpitations	R00.2	
780.03	Persistent Vegetative State	R40.3	
782.7	Petechiae	R23.3	
783.5	Polydipsia/Excess Thirst	R63.1	
788.42	Polyuria	R38.5	
784.91	Postnasal Drip	R09.82	
781.92	Posture, Abnormal	R29.3	

16. Symptoms, Signs, and Ill-defined Conditions *(cont)*

ICD-9-CM		ICD-10-CM	
791.0	Proteinuria	R80.9	
786.31	Pulmonary Hemorrhage, Acute Idiopathic in Infants >28 Days	R04.81	
782.1	*Rash*	R21	
788.0	Renal Colic	N23	
799.1	Respiratory Arrest	R09.2	
786.9	*Respiratory Complaint/Sx Breath-holding Spells*	R06.89	
790.1	Sedimentation Rate, Elevated	R70.0	
780.39	Seizure/Convulsions	R56.9	
780.32	Seizure, Febrile, Complex	R56.01	
780.31	Seizure, Febrile, Simple	R56.00	
780.33	Seizure, Post-traumatic	R56.1	
785.51	Shock, Cardiogenic	R57.0	
785.50	Shock, Nontraumatic	R57.9	
785.52	Shock, Septic add 995.92 if organ dysfunction present	R65.21*	Sepsis, Severe, w/ Septic Shock
783.43	Short Stature	R62.52	
786.05	Shortness of Breath	R06.02	
782.2	*Skin Mass/Lump/Nodule*	R22.-	by site
780.50	Sleep Disturbance	G47.9	
784.59	Speech Disturbance	R47.89	
789.2	Splenomegaly	R16.1	
792.1	*Stool, Abnormal*	R19.5	
786.1	Stridor	R06.1	
798.0	Sudden Infant Death Syndrome	R99	
780.2	Syncope/Fainting	R55	
785.0	Tachycardia	R00.0	
786.06	Tachypnea	R06.82	
795.52	TB Cellular Immunity Test, Nonspecific Reaction w/o Active TB	R76.12	
795.51	TB Skin Test Positive w/o Active TB	R76.11	

ICD-9-CM		ICD-10-CM
787.99	Tenesmus (Rectal)	R19.8
784.99	*Throat/Mouth Complaints/Sx*	R06.89
	Halitosis	R19.6
	Mouth Breathing	R06.5
784.1	Throat Pain	R07.0
781.93	Torticollis, Ocular	R29.891
781.0	Tremor	R25.1
780.09	Unconsciousness/Stupor	R40.1
783.22	Underweight	R63.6
	add code for BMI if known	Z68.-
788.7	Urethral Discharge	R36.9
788.9	*Urinary Complaints/Sx*	R39.89
788.41	Urinary Frequency	R35.0
788.64	Urinary Hesitancy	R39.11
788.30	Urinary Incontinence	R32
788.63	Urinary Urgency	R39.15
780.4	Vertigo (Dizziness)	R42
787.03	Vomiting (Alone)	R11.11
787.04	Vomiting, Bilious	R11.14
783.1	Weight Gain, Abnormal	R63.5
783.21	Weight Loss, Abnormal	R63.4
	add code for BMI if known	Z68.-
786.07	Wheezing	R06.2
793.19	X-ray, Chest, Nonspecific (Abnormal)	R91.8
793.7	X-ray, Musculoskeletal, Nonspecific (Abnormal)	R93.7
793.2	X-ray or Echocardiogram, Cardiac, Nonspecific (Abnormal)	R93.1
793.6	X-ray or Ultrasound, Abdominal, Nonspecific (Abnormal)	R93.5
793.0	X-ray or Ultrasound, Head/Skull, Nonspecific (Abnormal)	R93.0

16. Symptoms, Signs, and Ill-defined Conditions *(cont)*

ICD-9-CM		ICD-10-CM	
Other Related Diagnoses			
682.9	*Abscess/Lymphangitis, Unspec*	**LØ3.91**	
995.2Ø	Adverse Effect, Medication, Unspec	**T5Ø.9Ø5√**	
995.3	Allergic Reaction, Non-medication	**T78.3XX√**	
285.9	*Anemia*	**D64.9**	
427.9	*Arrhythmia, Cardiac*	**I49.9**	
716.9Ø	*Arthritis, Unspec*	**M12.9**	
716.1Ø	*Arthropathy, Traumatic*	**M12.5Ø**	
611.79	*Breast Problems*	**N64.59**	
459.9	*Cardiovascular Disease, Unspec*	**I99.9**	
682.9	*Cellulitis, Unspec*	**LØ3.9Ø**	
692.9	*Dermatitis, Contact, Unspec*	**L23.9**	
719.7	Difficulty Walking/Limp	**R26.2**	
995.27	Drug Allergy/Hypersensitivity	**T5Ø.995√**	
779.34	Failure to Thrive in Newborn	**P92.6**	
564.9	*Functional Disorder of Intestine*	**K59.9**	
V62.85	Homicidal Ideation	**R45.85**	
3Ø6.1	Hyperventilation, Psychogenic	**F45.8**	
536.8	Indigestion/Dyspepsia	**K3Ø**	
56Ø.9	*Intestinal Obstruction*	**K56.6Ø**	
579.8	*Milk/Formula Intolerance*	**K9Ø.4**	
313.1	*Misery/Unhappiness*	**F93.8**	
729.82	Muscle Cramps	**R25.2**	
728.85	Muscle Spasm	**M62.838**	
728.87	Muscle Weakness	**M62.81**	
729.1	Myalgia/Myositis	**M79.1**	Myalgia
		M6Ø.9	Myositis, Unspec
7Ø3.8	Nail Abnormalities/Diseases	**L6Ø.8**	
	Onycholysis	**L6Ø.1**	
358.9	*Neuromuscular Disorder*	**G7Ø.9**	
528.9	*Oral Complaints/Sx*	**K13.7-**	
388.7Ø	*Otalgia (Earache)*	**H92.Ø¤**	

ICD-9-CM		ICD-10-CM
338.11	Pain, Acute Due to Trauma	G89.11
338.18	Pain, Acute, Postoperative	G89.18
719.47	Pain, Ankle	M25.579∞
724.5	Pain, Back	M25.529∞
719.45	Pain, Hip	M25.559∞
719.46	Pain, Knee	M25.569∞
729.5	Pain, Limb Non-joint Pain in Extremity, Hand, Foot	M79.603∞ Pain in Arm, Unspec M79.606∞ Pain in Leg, Unspec M79.609 Pain in Unspec Limb
338.3	Pain, Neoplasm Related	G89.3
338.19	Pain, Other Acute	R52
719.43	Pain, Wrist	M25.539∞
521.89	Poor Dentition	K03.89
698.9	*Pruritus/Itch*	L29.9
345.90	*Seizure Disorder*	G40.901 w/ Status Epilepticus G40.909 w/o Status Epilepticus
345.91	*Seizure Disorder, Poorly Controlled*	G40.911 w/ Status Epilepticus G40.919 w/o Status Epilepticus
998.02	Shock, Septic Postoperative* add 995.92 if organ dysfunction present	T81.12X√
958.4	Shock, Traumatic	T79.4XX√
686.9	Skin Infection, Unspec	L08.9
V62.84	Suicide Attempt/Ideation/Risk	T14.91 Suicide Attempt R45.85 Suicide Ideation
623.5	Vaginal Discharge, Noninfectious	N89.8
368.9	*Visual Disturbance*	H53.9
369.9	*Visual Impairment*	H54.7
569.87	Vomiting of Fecal Matter	R11.13
536.2	Vomiting, Persistent (Nonpregnancy)	R11.10

17. Injury and Poisoning

ICD-10-CM codes are not valid for use at the time of publication and should not be reported until the official implementation date set by the Centers for Medicare & Medicaid Services.

ICD-9-CM		ICD-10-CM	
965.4	Acetaminophen Ingestion+	T39.1X5√	Adverse Effect
	E850.4 Accidental	T39.1X1√	
	E950.0 Intentional	T39.1X2√	
995.20	Adverse Effect, Medication, Unspec	T50.905√	
995.7	Adverse Reaction, Food	T78.00X√	
995.1	Allergic Angioedema	T78.40X√	
995.3	Allergic Reaction	T78.3XX√	
969.72	Amphetamines Ingestion+	T43.625√	Adverse Effect
	E854.2 Accidental	T43.621√	
	E950.3 Intentional	T43.622√	
863.89	Anal Sphincter Tear, Traumatic	S36.899√	
995.0	Anaphylactic Reaction, Nonfood+	T78.2XX√	
999.41	Anaphylactic Reaction to Blood and Blood Products	T80.51X√+	
995.62	Anaphylactic Reaction to Crustaceans	T78.02X√	
995.68	Anaphylactic Reaction to Eggs	T78.08X√	
995.65	Anaphylactic Reaction to Fish	T78.03X√	
995.60	Anaphylactic Reaction to Food	T78.09X√	
995.66	Anaphylactic Reaction to Food Additives	T78.06X√	
995.63	Anaphylactic Reaction to Fruits and Vegetables	T78.04X√	
995.67	Anaphylactic Reaction to Milk Products	T78.07X√	
995.61	Anaphylactic Reaction to Peanuts	T78.01X√	
995.64	Anaphylactic Reaction to Tree Nuts and Seeds	T78.05X√	
999.42	Anaphylactic Reaction to Vaccination	T80.51X√	
995.1	Angioneurotic Edema	T78.40X√	
994.7	Asphyxiation/Strangulation+	T71.9xx√	

ICD-9-CM			ICD-10-CM	
967.0	Barbiturate Ingestion+		T42.3-√	
	E851	Accidental	T42.3X1√	
	E950.1	Intentional	T42.3X2√	
995.54	Battered Child Syndrome		T74.12X¤	Child Neglect, Confirmed
			T76.12X¤	Child Neglect, Suspected
969.4	Benzodiazepine Ingestion+		T42.4-√	
	E853.2	Accidental	T42.4X1√	
	E950.3	Intentional	T42.4X2√	
998.11	Bleeding, Post-procedure		T88.8XX√	defer to complication code from specific chapter to describe procedure
949.1	Burn, First Degree, Unspec Site		T30.0XX√	not for inpatient use
941.00	Burn, Head/Face/Neck, Unspec Degree		T20.00X+√	external cause code to identify source, place, and intent of burn
945.00	Burn, Lower Limb, Unspec Degree		T24.009+√	external cause code to identify source, place, and intent of burn
949.2	Burn, Second Degree, Unspec Site		T30.0XX√	not for inpatient use
949.3	Burn, Third Degree, Unspec Site		T30.0XX√	not for inpatient use
942.00	Burn, Trunk, Unspec Degree		T21.00X+√	external cause code to identify source, place, and intent of burn
949.0	Burn, Unspec Site/Degree		T30.0XX√	not for inpatient use
943.00	Burn, Upper Limb, Unspec Degree		T22.0000X+√	external cause code to identify source, place, and intent of burn
944.00	Burn, Wrist, Hand, Unspec Degree		T23.009+√	external cause code to identify source, place, and intent of burn
986	Carbon Monoxide Inhalation+		T58.94X√	specify source
	E868.8	Accidental	T58.91X√	Unspec Source
	E952.1	Intentional	T58.92X√	Unspec Source
851.80	Cerebral Laceration and Contusion		S06.330√	w/o LOC

17. Injury and Poisoning *(cont)*

ICD-9-CM		ICD-10-CM	
995.51	Child Abuse, Emotional/ Psychological+	T74.32X√	
995.55	Child Abuse, Infant+	T74.4XX√	
995.59	Child Abuse/Neglect, Multiple Forms+	T74.92X√	Child Neglect, Confirmed
		T76.92X√	Child Neglect, Suspected
995.54	Child Abuse, Physical+	T74.12X√	Child Neglect, Confirmed
		T76.12X√	Child Neglect, Suspected
995.53	Child Abuse, Sexual/Rape+	T74.22X√	Child Abuse, Sexual, Confirmed
		T76.22X√	Child Abuse, Sexual, Suspected
995.50	Child Abuse, Unspec	T74.92X√	Child Neglect, Confirmed
		T76.92X√	Child Neglect, Suspected
995.52	Child Neglect (Nutritional)	T74.02X√	Child Neglect, Confirmed
		T76.02X√	Child Neglect, Suspected
970.8	Cocaine Ingestion+	T40.5X5√	Adverse Effect
	E854.3 Accidental	T40.5X1√	
	E950.4 Intentional	T40.5X2√	
850.5	Concussion w/ LOC, Unspec Duration	S06.0X9√	
850.0	Concussion w/o LOC	S06.0X0√	
924.9	*Contusion*	T14.8	
922.31	Contusion, Back	S30.0XX√	
922.32	Contusion, Buttock	S30.0XX√	
922.33	Contusion, Interscapular	S20.229√	
918.1	Corneal Abrasion	S05.02X√	Left Eye
		S05.01X√	Right Eye
		S05.00X√	Unspec Eye
929.0	*Crush Injury*	T07.-√	
927.3	Crushed Finger(s)	S67.10X√	Finger, Unspec
		S67.00X√	Thumb, Unspec
928.3	Crushed Toe(s)	S97.119√	Great Toe, Unspec
		S97.109√	Toes, Unspec

ICD-9-CM		ICD-10-CM	
972.1	Digoxin Ingestion+	T46.ØX5√	Adverse Effect
	E858.3 Accidental	T46.ØX1√	
	E95Ø.4 Intentional	T46.ØX2√	
834.ØØ	Dislocation, Finger, Closed	S36.259√	Finger, Unspec
		S36.1Ø6√∞	Thumb
754.3Ø	Dislocation, Hip, Unilateral, Congenital	Q65.ØØ∞	
836.5Ø	Dislocation, Knee, Closed	S83.1Ø5√	Dislocation, Knee, Left
		S83.1Ø4√	Dislocation, Knee, Right
		S83.1Ø6√	Dislocation, Knee, Unspec
836.3	Dislocation/Subluxation, Patella, Closed	S83.ØØ5√	Dislocation, Patella, Left
		S83.ØØ4√	Dislocation, Patella, Right
		S83.ØØ6√	Dislocation, Patella, Unspec
		S83.ØØ3√∞	Subluxation, Patella, Unspec
998.33	Disruption (Dehiscence) of Traumatic Injury Wound Repair	T81.33X√	
998.3Ø	Disruption of Wound	T81.3ØX√	
994.1	Drowning, Fatal or Nonfatal	T75.1XX√	
995.27	Drug Allergy/Hypersensitivity	T5Ø.995√	
977.9	Drug Ingestion, Unspec+	T5Ø.9Ø5√	Adverse Effect
	E858.9 Accidental	T5Ø.9Ø1√	
	E95Ø.4 Intentional	T5Ø.9Ø2	
994.8	Electric Shock	T75.4XX√	
994.9	Entrapped Digit w/o Other Injury Ring Stuck on Finger or Toe	T75.89X√	
999.82	Extravasation of Other Vesicant Agent	T8Ø.818√	
999.81	Extravasation of Vesicant Chemotherapy	T8Ø.81Ø	

17. Injury and Poisoning *(cont)*

ICD-9-CM		ICD-10-CM	
930.1	Foreign Body, Conjunctiva	T15.12X√	Left Eye
		T15.11X√	Right Eye
		T15.10X√	Unspec Eye
930.0	Foreign Body, Corneal	T15.02X√	Left Eye
		T15.01X√	Right Eye
		T15.00X√	Unspec Eye
931	Foreign Body, Ear	T16.2XX√	Foreign Body in Left Ear
		T16.1XX√	Foreign Body in Right Ear
		T16.9XX√	Foreign Body in Unspec Ear
935.1	Foreign Body, Esophagus	T18.1-±√	
938	Foreign Body, GI	T18.8XX√	
933.1	Foreign Body, Larynx (Choke)	T17.3-±√	
932	Foreign Body, Nose	T17.1XX√	
934.9	Foreign Body, Respiratory	T17.9-±√	
919.7	*Foreign Body, Skin w/ Infection*	T07.-√	
919.6	*Foreign Body, Skin w/o Infection*	T07.-√	
939.2	Foreign Body, Vagina	T19.2XX√	
824.8	Fx Ankle, Unspec, Closed	S82.899√	
801.01	Fx Base of Skull, Closed, w/o LOC/Bleed	S02.10X√	
805.00	Fx Cervical, Closed	S12.9XX√	
810.00	Fx Clavicle, Closed	S42.009√∞	
821.00	Fx Femur, Closed	S72.90X√∞	
823.41	Fx Fibula, Torus/Buckle	S82.829√∞ Lower End	
		S82.819√∞ Upper End	
816.00	Fx Finger(s)/Phalange(s) (Hand), Closed	S62.609√	Finger, Unspec
		S62.509√∞ Thumb	
825.20	Fx Foot/Metatarsal, Closed	S92.909√∞	
813.80	Fx Forearm, Unspec, Closed	S52.90X√∞	
815.00	Fx Hand/Metacarpal, Closed	S62.309√∞	
812.20	Fx Humerus, Closed	S42.309√∞	
802.20	Fx Mandible, Closed	S02.609√+ *associated intracranial injury S06.-*	
802.0	Fx Nasal Bone, Closed	S02.2XX√	
802.6	Fx Orbit (Blowout), Closed	S02.3XX√	

ICD-9-CM		ICD-10-CM	
808.8	Fx Pelvis, Unspec, Closed	S32.9XX√	
813.45	Fx Radius, Torus/Buckle	S52.119√∞	
813.47	Fx Radius/Ulna, Torus/Buckle	S52.129√∞ Radius, Lower End, Torus	
		S52.119√∞ Radius, Upper End, Torus	
		S52.629√∞ Ulna, Lower End, Torus	
		S52.009√∞ Ulna, Upper End, Torus	
807.00	Fx Rib(s), Closed	S22.39X√∞	
805.6	Fx Sacrum/Coccyx, Closed	S32.10X√	Sacrum
		S32.2XX√	Coccyx
800.01	Fx Skull, Closed, w/o LOC/Bleed	S02.0XX√	
823.80	Fx Tibia, Closed	S82.209√∞	
823.40	Fx Tibia, Torus/Buckle	See S82.319 and S82.169 Below	
823.82	Fx Tibia/Fibula, Closed	S82.209√∞ Tibia	
		S82.409√∞ Fibula	
823.42	Fx Tibia/Fibula, Torus/Buckle	S82.319√∞ Tibia, Lower End, Torus	
		S82.169√∞ Tibia, Upper End, Torus	
		S82.829√∞ Fibula, Lower End, Torus	
		S82.819√∞ Fibula, Upper End, Torus	
826.0	Fx Toe(s)/Phalange(s) (Foot), Closed	S92.406√	Great Toe, Unspec
		S92.506√	Lesser Toe(s), Unspec
813.46	Fx Ulna, Torus/Buckle	See S52.- Above	
814.00	Fx Wrist/Carpal, Closed	S92.109√∞	
987.1	Gasoline Inhalation	T59.894√	Undetermined
	E869.8 Accidental	T59.891√	
	E952.8 Intentional	T59.892√	
989.89	*Glue Sniffing+*	T52.8X1√	Accidental Poisoning
	E950.9 Intentional	T52.8X2√	Intentional
959.01	Head Injury w/o LOC	S09.8XX√	Head Injury, Other Specified
		S09.90X√	Head Injury, Unspec
992.2	Heat Cramps	T67.2XX√	
992.5	Heat Exhaustion	T67.3XX√	
992.6	Heat Fatigue	T67.6XX√	
992.0	Heat Stroke	T67.0XX√	

17. Injury and Poisoning *(cont)*

ICD-9-CM		ICD-10-CM	
981	Hydrocarbon Ingestion+	T52.ØX4√	Undetermined
	E862.1 Accidental	T52.ØX1√	
	E95Ø.9 Intentional	T52.ØX2√	
999.9	*Immunization Complication/ Reaction* add E879.8 as secondary code	T8Ø.62X√	
996.62	Infection Due to Arterial, Dialysis, or Peripheral Venous Vascular Device or Catheter	T82.7XX√	
999.31	Infection Due to Central Venous Catheter (PICC, Hickman)	T8Ø.219√	
999.39	Infection Following Other Infusion	T8Ø.29X√	
999.33	Infection of Central Venous Catheter Site	T8Ø.212√	
844.9	Injury, Knee Ligament	S83.9ØX√∞	
84Ø.4	Injury, Rotator Cuff	S43.429√∞	
919.5	*Insect Bite w/ Infection*	TØ7.-√	
919.4	*Insect Bite w/o Infection*	TØ7.-√	
869.Ø	*Internal Injury/Blunt Trauma*	S36.9ØX√	
853.ØØ	*Intracranial Hemorrhage, Traumatic*	SØ6.36Ø√	w/o LOC
964.Ø	Iron Ingestion+	T45.4X4√	Adverse Effect
	E858.2 Accidental	T45.4X1√	
	E95Ø.4 Intentional	T45.4X2√	
88Ø.Ø2	Laceration/Bite/Puncture, Axillae	S41.Ø19√	Laceration, Axillae, Unspec Side
		S41.Ø59√	Bite, Open, Axillae, Unspec Side
		S41.Ø39√	Puncture, Axillae, Unspec Side
873.4Ø	*Laceration/Bite/Puncture, Face*	SØ1.91X√	Laceration Unspec Part of Head
		SØ1.95X√	Bite, Open, Unspec Part of Head
		SØ1.93X√	Puncture, Unspec Part of Head

ICD-9-CM		ICD-10-CM	
883.0	Laceration/Bite/Puncture, Finger(s)	S61.219√	Laceration, Unspec Finger, w/o Nail Damage
		S61.259√	Bite, Open, Unspec Finger, w/o Nail Damage
		S61.239√	Puncture, Unspec Finger, w/o Nail Damage
892.0	Laceration/Bite/Puncture, Foot	S91.319√	Laceration, Unspec Foot
		S91.359√	Bite, Open, Unspec Foot
		S91.339√	Puncture, Unspec Foot
882.0	Laceration/Bite/Puncture, Hand	S61.419√	Laceration, Unspec Hand
		S61.459√	Bite, Open, Unspec Hand
		S61.439√	Puncture, Unspec Hand
894.0	Laceration/Bite/Puncture, Lower Extremity	S81.819√	Laceration, Unspec Lower Leg
		S81.859√	Bite, Open, Unspec Lower Leg
		S81.839√	Puncture, Unspec, Lower Leg
874.8	Laceration/Bite/Puncture, Neck	S11.91X√	Laceration, Unspec Part of Neck
		S11.95X√	Bite, Open, Unspec Part of Neck
		S11.93X√	Puncture, Unspec Part of Neck
873.0	Laceration/Bite/Puncture, Scalp	S01.01X√	Laceration, Scalp
		S01.05X√	Bite, Open, Scalp
		S01.03X√	Puncture, Scalp
893.0	Laceration/Bite/Puncture, Toe(s)	S91.119√	Laceration, Unspec Toe, w/o Nail Damage
		S91.159√	Bite, Open, Unspec Toe, w/o Nail Damage
		S91.139√	Puncture, Unspec Toe, w/o Nail Damage
879.6	Laceration/Bite/Puncture, Trunk	S31.010√	Laceration, Trunk
		S31.050√	Bite, Open, Trunk
		S31.030√	Puncture, Trunk

17. Injury and Poisoning *(cont)*

ICD-9-CM		ICD-10-CM	
884.0	Laceration/Bite/Puncture, Upper Extremity	S41.119√	Laceration, Unspec Upper Extremity
		S41.159√	Bite, Open, Unspec Upper Extremity
		S41.139√	Puncture, Unspec Upper Extremity
872.00	Laceration, Ears	S01.312√	Laceration w/o Foreign Body of Left Ear
		S01.311√	Laceration w/o Foreign Body of Right Ear
		S01.319√	Laceration w/o Foreign Body of Unspec Ear
878.8	Laceration, External/Genitalia	S31.512√	Female
		S31.511√	Male
870.1	Laceration, Eyelid	S01.11X√	
873.43	Laceration, Lip	S01.511√	
873.60	Laceration, Mouth	S01.502√	
873.20	Laceration, Nose	S01.21X√	
873.74	Laceration, Tongue	S01.512√	
878.6	Laceration, Vaginal Tear (Traumatic)	S31.40X√	
984.9	Lead Poisoning	T56.0X4√	Undetermined
	E866.0 Accidental	T56.0X1√	
861.21	Lung Contusion	S27.322	Bilateral
		S27.321	Unilateral
		S27.329	Unspec
983.2	Lye Ingestion+	T54.3X4√	Undetermined
	E864.2 Accidental	T54.3X1√	
	E950.7 Intentional	T54.3X2√	
996.2	Malfunction CNS Shunt	T85.09X√	
969.73	Methylphenidate Ingestion+	T43.634√	Undetermined
	E854.2 Accidental	T43.631√	
	E950.3 Intentional	T43.632√	
994.6	Motion Sickness	T75.3XX√	identify vehicle or type of motion Y92.81-, Y93.5-
988.1	Mushroom Ingestion+	T62.0X4√	Undetermined
	E865.5 Accidental	T62.0X1√	
	E950.9 Intentional	T62.0X2√	

ICD-9-CM		ICD-10-CM	
998.83	Nonhealing Surgical Wound	T81.89X√	
832.2	Nursemaid Elbow	S53.033√∞	
989.3	Organophosphate Poison+	T60.0X4√	Undetermined
	E863.1 Accidental	T60.0X1√	
	E950.6 Intentional	T60.0X2√	
872.61	Perforated Eardrum, Traumatic	S09.22X√	Left Eardrum
		S09.21X√	Right Eardrum
		S09.20X√	Unspec Eardrum
966.1	Phenytoin Ingestion+	T42.0X4√	
	E855.0 Accidental	T42.0X1√	
	E950.4 Intentional	T42.0X2√	
997.32	Pneumonia, Post-procedural Aspiration	J95.89+	to identify disorder
860.0	Pneumothorax, Traumatic	S27.0XX√	
969.9	Psychotropic Agents Ingestion+	T43.94X√	Undetermined
	E855.9 Accidental	T43.91X√	
	E950.3 Intentional	T43.92X√	
866.00	Renal Contusion	S37.009√	
865.02	Ruptured Spleen	S36.030√	
965.1	Salicylate (ASA) Ingestion+	T39.094√	Undetermined
	E850.3 Accidental	T39.091√	
	E950.0 Intentional	T39.092√	
995.91	Sepsis* Systemic Inflammatory Response Syndrome (SIRS) w/o Organ Dysfunction	A41.9	
995.92	Sepsis, Severe* Systemic Inflammatory Response Syndrome (SIRS) w/o Organ Dysfunction	R65.20*	Sepsis
999.31	Septicemia Due to Central Venous Catheter (PICC, Hickman)	T80.219	
999.59	Serum Sickness	T80.69X√	
995.55	Shaken Baby Syndrome	T74.4XX√	

17. Injury and Poisoning *(cont)*

ICD-9-CM		ICD-10-CM	
998.00	Shock, Postoperative	T81.10X√	
998.02	Shock, Septic Postoperative* add 995.92 if organ dysfunction present	T81.12X√	
958.4	Shock, Traumatic	T79.4XX√	
952.9	*Spinal Cord Injury*	S14.109√	Cervical
		S34.109√	Lumbar
		S34.139√	Sacrum
		S24.109√	Thoracic
845.00	Sprain/Strain, Ankle	S93.409√∞	
841.9	Sprain/Strain, Elbow	S53.409√∞	
845.10	Sprain/Strain, Foot/Toe	S93.609√∞	Foot
		S93.503√∞	Great Toe
		S93.506√∞	Other Unspec Toe
842.10	Sprain/Strain, Hand/Finger	S63.90X√∞	Hand
		S63.619√∞	Other Unspec Finger
		S63.609√∞	Thumb
844.9	Sprain/Strain, Knee	S83.90X√∞	
846.0	Sprain/Strain, Lumbosacral	S33.8XX√	
847.0	Sprain/Strain, Neck/Whiplash	S13.4XX√	
842.00	Sprain/Strain, Wrist	S63.509√∞	
958.7	SQ Emphysema, Traumatic	T79.7XX√	
848.1	Strain, TMJ	S03.4XX√	
852.00	*Subarachnoid Bleed, Traumatic*	S06.6X9√	w/ LOC Unspec Duration
		S06.6X0√	w/o LOC
852.20	*Subdural Hemorrhage, Traumatic*	S06.5X9√	w/ LOC Unspec Duration
		S06.5X0√	w/o LOC
927.3	Subungual Hematoma of Finger	S67.10X√	Finger, Unspec
		S67.00X√	Thumb, Unspec
928.3	Subungual Hematoma of Toe	S97.119√	Great Toe, Unspec
		S97.109√	Toes, Unspec
919.8	*Superficial Injury, Unspec w/o Infection*	T07.-√	
995.94	Systemic Inflammatory Response Syndrome (SIRS), Noninfectious w/ Organ Dysfunction*	R65.11*+	*underlying condition acute organ dysfunction*

ICD-9-CM		ICD-10-CM
995.93	Systemic Inflammatory Response Syndrome (SIRS), Noninfectious w/o Organ Dysfunction*	R65.10* *underlying condition*
975.7	Theophylline Ingestion+	T48.6X4√ Undetermined
	E858.6 Accidental	T48.6X1√
	E950.4 Intentional	T48.6X2√
873.63	Tooth, Broken w/o Complication	S02.5XX√
989.89	*Toxic Ingestion (Nonmedicinal)+*	T64.94X√
	E866.8 Accidental	T65.91X√
	E950.9 Intentional	T65.92X√
999.80	*Transfusion Reaction*	T80.92X√
999.84	*Transfusion Reaction, Acute Hemolytic*	T80.910√
999.85	*Transfusion Reaction, Delayed Hemolytic*	T80.911√
996.80	Transplant Complication	T86.90X√
996.85	Transplant Failure/Rejection, Bone Marrow	T86.02X√ Failure / T86.01X√ Rejection
996.83	Transplant Failure/Rejection, Heart	T86.22X√ Failure / T86.21X√ Rejection
996.81	Transplant Failure/Rejection, Kidney	T86.12X√ Failure / T86.11X√ Rejection
996.82	Transplant Failure/Rejection, Liver	T86.42X√ Failure / T86.41X√ Rejection
996.84	Transplant Failure/Rejection, Lung	T86.811√ Failure / T86.810√ Rejection
996.88	Transplant Failure/Rejection, Stem Cell	T86.5XX√
959.1	Trauma, GU/Pelvis/Perineum	S39.848√ GU/Perineum / S39.83X√ Pelvis
969.05	Tricyclic Ingestion+	T43.014√ Undetermined
	E854.0 Accidental	T43.011√
	E950.3 Intentional	T43.012√
999.0	Vaccinia	T88.1XX√

17. Injury and Poisoning *(cont)*

ICD-9-CM		ICD-10-CM	
989.5	Venomous Bite	T63.91X√	Venomous Bite, Unspec Animal, Accidental
	Bee	T63.441√	Accidental
	Jellyfish	T63.621√	Accidental
	Snake	T63.001√	Snake, Unspec, Accidental
	Spider	T63.301√	Spider, Unspec, Accidental
	Tick	T63.481√	
997.31	Ventilator-Associated Pneumonia	J95.851+	*to identify organism*

Other Related Diagnoses			
348.82	Brain Death	G93.82	
521.81	Cracked Tooth	K03.81	
V15.86	Exposure (or Suspected) to Lead	Z77.011	
767.2	Fx Clavicle, Newborn	P13.4	
767.3	Fx Skull, Newborn/Molded Head	P13.0	
V15.86	Lead Exposure, Hx of	Z77.011	
790.6	Lead Test, Positive, Nonspecific	R78.71	
518.1	Mediastinal Air/ Pneumomediastinum	J98.2	
785.52	Shock, Septic add 995.92 if organ dysfunction present	R65.21*	Sepsis, Severe, w/ Septic Shock
733.94	Stress Fx, Metatarsals	M84.375√	Left Foot
		M84.374√	Right Foot
		M84.376√	Unspec Foot
733.95	Stress Fx, Other Bone	M84.38X√	
733.93	Stress Fx, Tibia or Fibula	M84.362√	Left Tibia
		M84.361√	Right Tibia
		M84.364√	Left Fibula
		M84.363√	Right Fibula
		M84.369√	Unspec Tibia or Fibula
623.4	Vaginal Tear (Nontraumatic)	N89.8	

V Codes: Classification of Factors Influencing Health Status and Contact With Health Services

ICD-10-CM codes are not valid for use at the time of publication and should not be reported until the official implementation date set by the Centers for Medicare & Medicaid Services.

ICD-9-CM		ICD-10-CM	
Outcome of Delivery			
V37.01	Liveborn, Multiple, by Cesarean	Z38.64	Quadruplet
		Z38.62	Triplet
V37.00	Liveborn, Multiple, in Hospital	Z38.63	Quadruplet
		Z38.62	Triplet
V30.01	Liveborn, Single, by Cesarean	Z38.01	
V30.00	Liveborn, Single, in Hospital	Z38.00	
V30.1	Liveborn, Single, Out of Hospital	Z38.1	
V31.01	Liveborn, Twins, by Cesarean	Z38.31	
V31.00	Liveborn, Twins, in Hospital	Z38.30	
V31.1	Liveborn, Twins, Out of Hospital	Z38.4	

Physician Care Visits: Encounters (May Be Used as Primary Visit Code)		
V70.3	Administrative Medical Exam	Z02.89
	Adoption Exam	Z02.82
	Camp Exam	Z02.89
	Sports Exam	Z02.5
	School Admission Exam	Z02.0
V72.7	Allergy Testing	Z01.82
V49.83	Awaiting Organ Transplant	Z76.82
V58.11	Chemotherapy, Encounter for	Z51.11
V58.49	Circumcision Care	Z48.89
V50.2	Circumcision, Encounter for	Z41.2
V25.03	Contraception, Emergency Counseling and Prescription	Z30.012
V25.02	Contraception Initiation, IUD	Z30.014
V25.01	Contraception Initiation, Oral	Z30.011
V25.40	*Contraception Surveillance*	Z30.40

V Codes: Classification of Factors Influencing Health Status and Contact With Health Services *(cont)*

ICD-9-CM		ICD-10-CM	
Physician Care Visits: Encounters (May Be Used as Primary Visit Code) *(cont)*			
V25.42	Contraceptive Monitoring, IUD includes removal and reinsertion	**Z30.430**	Encounter for Insertion of IUD
		Z30.433	Encounter for Removal and Reinsertion of IUD
		Z30.432	Encounter for Removal of IUD
		Z30.431	Routine Checking of IUD
V25.41	Contraceptive Monitoring, Oral includes repeat prescription	**Z30.41**	
V65.3	Diet Surveillance and Counseling	**Z71.3+**	*underlying medical condition and BMI if known Z68.-*
V68.01	Disability Exam	**Z02.71**	
V58.30	Dressing and Wound Care, Nonsurgical	**Z48.00**	
V58.31	Dressing and Wound Care, Surgical	**Z48.01**	
V70.5	Exam for Specific Groups	**Z02.89**	
	Preschool Children	**Z02.0**	
	Schoolchildren/Students	**Z02.0**	
V67.59	Follow-up Exam, After Treatment Asthma Exacerbation Course (Short) of Therapy (Antibiotic) STD	**Z09**	
V67.01	Follow-up Exam, Pap Smear	**Z08**	
V72.32	Follow-up Exam, Pap Smear to Confirm Findings of Recent Normal Smear	**Z01.42**	Following Initial Abnormal Smear
V58.89	Follow-up Exam/Recheck, Unspec	**Z51.89**	
V55.1	Gastrostomy Tube Problem Clogged Dislodged	**Z43.1**	
V70.0	General Medical Exam (Not Child)	**Z00.01+**	w/ Abnormal Findings *to identify findings*
		Z00.00	w/o Abnormal Findings

ICD-9-CM		ICD-10-CM	
V72.31	Gynecological Exam, Routine	Z01.411+	w/ Abnormal Findings *to identify findings*
		Z01.419	w/o Abnormal Findings
V20.2	Health Check for Infant/Child Developmental Evaluation Routine Immunizations Well-Child Care for Child >28 Days of Age (includes routine vision and hearing screens) add code(s) for special screening exams	Z00.121+	w/ Abnormal Findings *to identify findings*
		Z00.129	w/o Abnormal Findings
V20.31	Health Check for Newborn <8 Days of Age	Z00.110	
V20.32	Health Check for Newborn 8–28 Days of Age Newborn Weight Check	Z00.111	
V72.12	Hearing Conservation and Treatment	Z01.12	
V72.11	Hearing Exam After Failed Hearing Screen	Z01.110	
V72.19	Hearing Exam, Other not part of a routine or general exam	Z01.10	Hearing Exam, w/o Abnormal Findings
V62.85	Homicidal Ideation	R45.85	
V68.09	Issue Medical Certification (Only)	Z02.79	
V68.1	Issue Repeat Prescription (Only) excludes contraceptives	Z76.0	
V58.62	Long-term (Current) Use of Antibiotics	Z79.2	
V58.66	Long-term (Current) Use of Aspirin	Z79.82	
V58.67	Long-term (Current) Use of Insulin	Z79.4	
V58.64	Long-term (Current) Use of Nonsteroidal Anti-inflammatories	Z79.1	
V58.69	Long-term (Current) Use of Other (High-risk) Medications Anticonvulsants Anti-reflux Drugs Chemotherapy	Z79.899	

V Codes: Classification of Factors Influencing Health Status and Contact With Health Services *(cont)*

ICD-9-CM		ICD-10-CM	
Physician Care Visits: Encounters (May Be Used as Primary Visit Code) *(cont)*			
V58.65	Long-term (Current) Use of Steroids	Z79.51	Inhaled Steroids
		Z79.52	Systemic Steroids
V70.4	Medicolegal Exam	Z02.89	
V65.11	Pre-birth Visit by Expectant Parent(s) Pre-adoption Visit for Adoptive Parent(s)	Z76.81	
V72.41	Pregnancy Test, Negative	Z32.02	
V72.42	Pregnancy Test, Positive	Z32.01	
V72.40	Pregnancy Test, Pregnancy Unconfirmed	Z32.00	
V22.2	Pregnant	Z33.1	
V72.83	Preoperative General Exam	Z01.818	
V58.0	Radiation Therapy, Encounter for	Z51.0	
V68.81	Referral of Patient (Only)	Z04.9	
V90.31	Retained Animal Quills or Spines	Z18.31	
V90.9	Retained Foreign Body	Z18.9	
V90.89	Retained Foreign Body, Other Specified	Z18.89	
V90.81	Retained Glass Fragments	Z18.81	
V90.11	Retained Magnetic Metal Fragments	Z18.11	
V90.10	Retained Metal Fragments, Unspec	Z18.10	
V90.12	Retained Nonmagnetic Metal Fragments	Z18.12	
V90.39	Retained Other Organic Fragments	Z18.39	
V90.2	Retained Plastic Fragments	Z18.2	
V90.83	Retained Stone or Crystalline Fragments	Z18.83	
V90.32	Retained Tooth	Z18.32	
V90.33	Retained Wood Fragments	Z18.33	
V62.84	Suicide Attempt/Ideation/Risk	T14.91	Suicide Attempt
		R45.85	Suicide Ideation

ICD-9-CM		ICD-10-CM	
V58.32	Suture/Staple Removal	Z48.02	
V58.83	Therapeutic Drug Monitoring	Z51.81+	*any long-term (current) drug therapy Z79.-*
V72.Ø	Vision Exam, Special not part of a routine or general exam	ZØ1.Ø1	w/ Abnormal Findings
		ZØ1.ØØ	w/o Abnormal Findings

Physician Care Visits With No Findings (May Be Used as Primary Visit Code)		
V2Ø.Ø	Exam Foundling/Abandoned Child	Z76.1
V71.4	Obs Following Accident Exam After Vehicle Accident	ZØ4.3
V71.3	Obs Following Accident at Work (School)	ZØ4.2
V71.6	Obs Following Inflicted Injury Exam of Assault Victim	ZØ4.8
V71.5	Obs for Alleged Rape Exam for Alleged Rape	ZØ4.42
V71.Ø2	Obs for Antisocial Behavior, Nonpsychiatric	ZØ3.89
V29.3	Obs for Genetic or Metabolic Condition, Newborn	PØØ.89
V29.8	Obs for Other Suspected Condition, Newborn	PØØ.89
V29.2	Obs for Respiratory Condition, Newborn Evaluation for Neonatal Apnea	PØØ.3
V71.82	Obs for Suspected Anthrax Exposure	ZØ3.81Ø
V71.83	Obs for Suspected Biologic Agent Exposure	ZØ3.818
V71.7	Obs for Suspected Cardiovascular Disease	ZØ3.89
V29.1	Obs for Suspected CNS Disease, Newborn Evaluation for Neonatal Seizure	PØØ.89

V Codes: Classification of Factors Influencing Health Status and Contact With Health Services *(cont)*

ICD-9-CM		ICD-10-CM
Physician Care Visits With No Findings (May Be Used as Primary Visit Code) *(cont)*		
V71.89	Obs for Suspected Condition Evaluation for Foreign Body Ingestion Evaluation for Meningitis Evaluation for Septicemia Evaluation for Surgical Condition	Z03.89
V29.0	Obs for Suspected Infection, Newborn Evaluation for Sepsis/Infection	P00.2
V71.1	Obs for Suspected Malignant Neoplasm	Z03.89
V71.09	Obs for Suspected Mental Condition	Z03.89
V71.81	Obs for Suspected Neglect and Abuse Exam for Alleged Child Abuse/ Neglect	Z04.72
V71.2	Obs for Suspected TB	Z03.89
V71.9	Obs for Unspec Suspected Condition	Z04.9
V89.03	Suspected Fetal Anomaly Not Found	Z03.73
V89.04	Suspected Problem w/ Fetal Growth Not Found	Z03.74

ICD-9-CM		ICD-10-CM
Physician Care Visits: Counseling (May Be Used as Primary Visit Code)		
V65.40	Child/Adolescent Conference	Z71.89
V65.43	Counsel Injury Prevention	Z71.89
V61.10	Counsel Marital/Partner Problem	Z71.89
V61.24	Counsel Parent-Adopted Child Problem	Z62.821
V61.23	Counsel Parent-Biological Child Problem	Z62.820
V61.25	Counsel Parent (Guardian)- Foster Child Problem	Z62.822
V61.22	Counsel Perpetrator Parental Child Abuse	Z69.011

ICD-9-CM		ICD-10-CM	
V62.83	Counsel Perpetrator Sexual Abuse	**Z69.82**	
V61.12	Counsel Perpetrator Spousal Abuse	**Z69.12**	
V61.8	Counsel Sibling Relationship Problem	**Z62.891**	
V65.45	Counsel STD Prevention	**Z71.89**	
V65.42	Counsel Substance Abuse	**Z71.4Ø**	
		Z71.6+	Counsel Tobacco *for nicotine dependence F17.-*
V61.21	Counsel Victim Child Abuse	**Z69.Ø1Ø**	
V61.11	Counsel Victim Spousal Abuse	**Z69.11**	
V65.3	Diet Surveillance and Counseling	**Z71.3+**	*underlying medical condition and BMI if known Z68.-*
V65.19	Family (Extended) Conference	**Z71.Ø**	
V25.Ø9	Family Planning Advice	**Z3Ø.Ø9**	
V26.33	Genetic Counseling	**Z31.5**	
V65.4Ø	Health Counseling/Education	**Z71.9**	
V65.44	HIV Counseling	**Z71.7**	
V25.Ø4	*Natural Family Planning Counseling to Avoid Pregnancy*	**Z3Ø.Ø2**	
V65.49	Parent Conference	**Z71.89**	
V26.49	Pregnancy Counseling	**Z31.69**	

Special Screening Exams for: (Supplementary Code)			
V82.1	Arthritis	**Z13.828**	
V74.8	Bacterial and Spirochetal Disease Pertussis Tetanus	**Z11.2**	Bacterial Pertussis Tetanus
		Z11.8	Spirochetal
V74.5	Bacterial and Spirochetal Disease, STD	**Z11.3**	
V81.2	Cardiovascular Disease	**Z13.6**	
V73.88	Chlamydial Disease	**Z11.8**	
V77.91	Cholesterol Screening	**Z13.22Ø**	

V Codes: Classification of Factors Influencing Health Status and Contact With Health Services *(cont)*

ICD-9-CM		ICD-10-CM	
Special Screening Exams for: (Supplementary Code) *(cont)*			
V82.89	Congenital Anomaly Nongenetic Testing	**Z13.89**	
V82.3	Congenital Hip Dislocation	**Z13.828**	
V77.6	Cystic Fibrosis	**Z13.228**	
V79.3	Developmental Delay, Early Childhood	**Z13.4**	excludes routine development testing of infant or child Z00.1-
V77.1	Diabetes Mellitus	**Z13.1**	
V77.99	*Endocrine, Nutritional, Metabolic, and Immune Disease, Unspec*	**Z13.29**	Endocrine
		Z13.21	Nutritional
		Z13.228	Metabolic
		Z13.0	Immune
V82.71	Genetic Disease Carrier Testing	**Z13.71**	
V82.79	Genetic Testing, Other	**Z13.79**	
V73.81	HPV	**Z11.51**	
V77.7	*Inborn Errors of Metabolism*	**Z13.228**	
V75.9	*Infectious Disease, Unspec*	**Z11.9**	
V75.7	Intestinal Helminthiasis	**Z11.6**	
V78.0	Iron Deficiency Anemia	**Z13.0**	
V82.5	Lead Poisoning	**Z13.88**	
V75.1	Malaria	**Z11.8**	
V73.2	Measles	**Z11.59**	
V79.9	*Mental Disorder, Unspec*	**Z13.89**	
V75.4	Mycotic Infection	**Z11.8**	
V76.81	Neoplasm, Nervous System	**Z12.82**	
V76.89	Neoplasm, Other Blood/Lymph Renal	**Z12.89**	
V76.9	*Neoplasm, Unspec*	**Z13.9**	
V80.09	Neurologic Condition	**Z13.858**	
V77.3	Phenylketonuria	**Z13.228**	
V81.4	Respiratory Conditions	**Z13.83**	
V75.0	Rickettsial Disease	**Z11.8**	
V76.11	Screening Mammography, High-risk	**Z12.31**	

ICD-9-CM		ICD-10-CM
V78.2	Sickle Cell	Z13.0
V74.1	TB	Z11.1
V77.0	Thyroid Disorder	Z13.29
V80.01	Traumatic Brain Injury	Z13.850
V73.89	Viral, Other Specified Enterovirus Epstein-Barr Virus	Z11.59

Patient Needs at Time of Visit (Supplementary Code)		
V61.3	Aged (Older) Parents	Z63.79
V07.1	Allergy Desensitization	Z51.89
V66.7	End-of-Life Palliative Care*	Z51.5+ condition requiring care
V07.2	Prophylactic Immunotherapy	Z41.8
V06.1	Vaccination, DTP/DTaP/Tdap	Z23
V05.3	Vaccination, Hepatitis	Z23
V03.81	Vaccination, Hib	Z23
V04.89	Vaccination, HPV	Z23
V04.81	Vaccination, Influenza	Z23
V04.2	Vaccination, Measles	Z23
V03.89	Vaccination, Meningococcal	Z23
V06.4	Vaccination, MMR	Z23
V06.8	Vaccination, Other Combinations	Z23
V05.9	Vaccination, Other Single Disease	Z23
V03.89	Vaccination, Other Specified Bacteria	Z23
V04.89	Vaccination, Other Viral Disease	Z23
V03.82	Vaccination, Pneumococcus	Z23
V04.0	Vaccination, Polio	Z23
V04.89	Vaccination, Rotavirus	Z23
V04.82	Vaccination, RSV	Z23
V04.3	Vaccination, Rubella	Z23
V06.5	Vaccination, Td/DT	Z23
V03.7	Vaccination, Tetanus Toxoid	Z23
V05.4	Vaccination, Varicella	Z23

V Codes: Classification of Factors Influencing Health Status and Contact With Health Services (cont)

ICD-9-CM		ICD-10-CM
Conditions Affecting Health (Supplementary Code)		
V47.5	Absent Testicle	R68.89
V15.89	Adopted Infant/Child	Z91.89
V21.8	Advanced Bone Age	Z00.2
V61.41	Alcohol Abuse in Family	Z63.72
V15.03	Allergic to Eggs	Z91.012
V15.06	Allergic to Insects and Spiders	Z91.038
V15.07	Allergic to Latex	Z91.011
V15.02	Allergic to Milk Products	Z91.011
V14.5	Allergic to Narcotics	Z88.5
V14.1	Allergic to Other Antibiotics	Z88.1
V15.05	Allergic to Other Foods	Z91.018
V15.09	Allergic to Other Nonmedicinal Agents	Z91.048
V14.8	Allergic to Other Specific Medicinals	Z88.8
V15.01	Allergic to Peanuts	Z91.010
V14.0	Allergic to Penicillin	Z88.0
V15.04	Allergic to Seafood	Z91.013
V14.2	Allergic to Sulfa	Z88.2
V14.7	Allergic to Vaccine/Serum	Z88.7
V15.88	At Risk for Falling	Z97.81
V69.5	Behavioral Insomnia of Childhood	Z73.819
V40.39	Behavioral Problems	F69
V85.51	BMI <5% for Age	Z68.51
V85.52	BMI 5%–<85% for Age	Z68.52
V85.53	BMI 85%–<95% for Age	Z68.53
V85.54	BMI ≥95% for Age	Z68.54
V45.01	Cardiac Pacemaker Present	Z95.0
V83.81	Carrier, Cystic Fibrosis Gene	Z14.1
V02.7	Carrier, Gonorrhea	Z22.4
V83.01	Carrier, Hemophilia A, Asymptomatic	Z14.01

ICD-9-CM		ICD-10-CM	
V83.02	Carrier, Hemophilia A, Symptomatic	Z14.02	
V02.61	Carrier, Hepatitis B	Z22.51	
V02.62	Carrier, Hepatitis C	Z22.52	
V02.60	Carrier, Hepatitis Unspec	Z22.50	
V02.59	Carrier, Meningococcus or Other Specified Bacterial Disease	Z22.31	Carrier, Meningococcus
		Z22.8	Carrier, Other Specified
V02.54	Carrier, MRSA	Z22.322	
V02.53	Carrier, MSSA	Z22.321	
V83.89	Carrier, Other Genetic Condition	Z14.8	
V02.8	Carrier, Other STD	Z22.4	
V02.52	Carrier, Streptococcus, Not Group B	Z22.338	
V45.2	Cerebral VP/VA Shunt Present	Z98.2	
V15.83	Delinquent Immunizations	Z28.3	
V49.86	Do-Not-Resuscitate Status	Z66	
V09.1	Drug-resistant Infection, Cephalosporins/ß-Lactams	Z16.19	Cephalosporins
		Z16.10	Unspec ß-Lactams
V09.81	Drug-resistant Infection, Multiple Agents	Z16.24	
V09.0	Drug-resistant Infection, Penicillin, MRSA	Z16.11	
V09.90	*Drug-resistant Infection, Single Agent*	Z16.29	
V09.80	Drug-resistant Infection, Vancomycin	Z16.21	
V49.85	Dual Sensory Impairment Combined Visual-Hearing Impairment	Z73.82	
V60.2	Economic Problem/Poverty	Z59.5	
V62.3	Educational/Academic Problem	Z55.9	
V87.11	Exposure (or Suspected) to Aromatic Amines	Z77.020	
V87.01	Exposure (or Suspected) to Arsenic	Z77.010	

V Codes: Classification of Factors Influencing Health Status and Contact With Health Services *(cont)*

ICD-9-CM		ICD-10-CM
Conditions Affecting Health (Supplementary Code) *(cont)*		
V15.84	Exposure (or Suspected) to Asbestos	**Z77.090**
V87.12	Exposure (or Suspected) to Benzene	**Z77.021**
V15.86	Exposure (or Suspected) to Lead	**Z77.011**
V87.31	Exposure (or Suspected) to Mold	**Z77.120**
V87.19	Exposure (or Suspected) to Other Hazardous Aromatic Compounds	**Z77.028**
V87.09	Exposure (or Suspected) to Other Hazardous Metals	**Z77.018**
V87.2	Exposure (or Suspected) to Other Potentially Hazardous Chemicals	**Z77.098**
V87.39	Exposure (or Suspected) to Other Potentially Hazardous Substances	**Z77.29**
V15.85	Exposure (or Suspected) to Potentially Hazardous Body Fluids	**Z57.8**
V01.81	Exposure to Anthrax	**Z20.810**
V01.83	Exposure to E. coli	**Z20.01**
V01.84	Exposure to Meningococcus	**Z20.811**
V01.89	*Exposure to Other Communicable Disease*	**Z20.89**
V01.79	*Exposure to Other Viral Disease*	**Z20.828**
	Exposure to Hepatitis	**Z20.5**
	Exposure to HIV	**Z20.6**
V01.5	Exposure to Rabies	**Z20.3**
V01.4	Exposure to Rubella	**Z20.4**
V15.89	Exposure to Secondhand Smoke	**Z77.22**
E869.4	Exposure to Secondhand Smoke	
V01.6	Exposure to STD	**Z20.2**
V01.1	Exposure to TB	**Z20.1**
V01.71	Exposure to Varicella	**Z20.820**
V61.06	Family Disruption Due to Child in Foster Care or w/ Non-parental Family Member	**Z63.32**
V61.05	Family Disruption Due to Child in Welfare Custody	**Z63.32**

ICD-9-CM		ICD-10-CM	
V61.07	Family Disruption Due to Death of Family Member	Z63.4	
V61.03	Family Disruption Due to Divorce or Legal Separation	Z63.5	
V61.01	Family Disruption Due to Family Member on Military Deployment	Z63.31	
V61.08	Family Disruption Due to Other Extended Absence of Family Member	Z63.32	
V61.04	Family Disruption Due to Parent-Child Estrangement	Z63.8	
V61.02	Family Disruption Due to Return of Family Member From Military Deployment	Z63.8	
V61.09	Family Disruption, Other	Z63.8	
V60.81	Foster Care	Z62.21	
V69.3	Gambling Problem	Z72.6	
V44.1	Gastrostomy Present	Z93.1	
V41.2	Hearing Problem	H93.299	
V42.1	Heart Transplant Present	Z94.1	
V43.3	Heart Valve Present, Prosthesis	Z95.2	
V42.2	Heart Valve Present, Transplant	Z95.3	
V23.84	High-risk Pregnancy, Young Multigravida <16 Years of Age at Expected Delivery	O09.62±	
V23.83	High-risk Pregnancy, Young Primigravida <16 Years of Age at Expected Delivery	O09.61±	
		±For High-risk Pregnancy Codes, Use 6th Digit 1 = First Trimester; 2 = Second Trimester; 3 = Third Trimester; 9 = Unspec Trimester	
V69.2	High-risk Sexual Behavior	Z72.53	High-risk Bisexual Behavior
		Z72.51	High-risk Heterosexual Behavior
		Z72.52	High-risk Homosexual Behavior

V Codes: Classification of Factors Influencing Health Status and Contact With Health Services *(cont)*

ICD-9-CM		ICD-10-CM	
Conditions Affecting Health (Supplementary Code) *(cont)*			
VØ8	HIV Infection w/o Sx	Z21	
V6Ø.Ø	Homeless	Z59.Ø	
V6Ø.1	Inadequate Housing	Z59.1	
V69.1	Inappropriate Diet/Eating Habits	Z72.4	
V45.72	Intestine, Acquired Absence	Z9Ø.49	
V45.73	Kidney, Acquired Absence	Z9Ø.5	
V69.Ø	Lack of Physical Exercise	Z72.3	
V21.31	LBW, <5ØØ g	PØ7.Ø1	
V21.32	LBW, 5ØØ–999 g	PØ7.Ø2	Extremely LBW Newborn, 5ØØ-749 g
		PØ7.Ø3	Extremely LBW Newborn, 75Ø-999 g
V21.33	LBW, 1,ØØØ–1,499 g	PØ7.1-	See Prematurity
V21.34	LBW, 1,5ØØ–1,999 g	PØ7.1-	See Prematurity
V21.35	LBW, 2,ØØØ–2,5ØØ g	PØ7.1-	See Prematurity
V4Ø.Ø	Learning Problems	F81.9	
V63.1	Medical Services in Home Not Available	Z75.Ø	
V6Ø.4	No Household Member Able to Render Care	Z74.2	
V15.81	Noncompliance w/ Medical Care	Z91.19	
V45.12	Noncompliance w/ Renal Dialysis	Z91.15	
V49.87	Physical Restraints Status	Z78.1	
V45.89	Postoperative Status excludes transplants, prosthesis placement, removal of kidney and intestine, major organ and heart surgery	Z98.89	
V21.1	Puberty	ZØØ.3	
V21.Ø	Rapid Growth in Childhood Accelerated Growth Rate	ZØØ.2	
V45.11	Renal Dialysis Status	Z99.2	
V42.Ø	Renal Transplant Present	Z94.Ø	
V69.8	Self-damaging Behavior	Z72.89	

ICD-9-CM		ICD-10-CM
V62.4	Social Maladjustment Cultural Deprivation	Z60.3
V61.42	Substance Abuse in Family	Z63.72
V45.87	Transplanted Organ Removed	Z98.85
V15.83	Under-immunized	Z28.3
V64.01	Vaccination Not Given Due to Acute Illness	Z28.01
V64.04	Vaccination Not Given Due to Allergy to Vaccine or Component	Z28.04
V64.05	Vaccination Not Given Due to Caregiver Refusal	Z28.82
V64.02	Vaccination Not Given Due to Chronic Illness or Condition	Z28.02
V64.03	Vaccination Not Given Due to Immune-compromised State	Z28.03
V64.06	Vaccination Not Given Due to Patient Refusal	Z28.20
V64.07	Vaccination Not Given for Religious Reasons	Z28.1
V64.09	Vaccination Not Given, Other Reason	Z28.89
V64.08	Vaccination Not Given, Patient Had Disease Being Vaccinated Against	Z28.81
V64.00	Vaccination Not Given, Unspec Reason	Z28.9
V41.0	Visual Impairment Problem	H54.7
V40.31	Wandering in Conditions Classified Elsewhere*	Z91.83*

V Codes: Classification of Factors Influencing Health Status and Contact With Health Services *(cont)*

ICD-9-CM	ICD-10-CM
Past Medical History Affecting Health (History of:) (Supplementary Code)	
V13.81 Anaphylaxis, Hx of	**Z87.892**
V87.41 Antineoplastic Chemotherapy, Hx of	**Z92.21**
V12.3 Blood Disorders, Hx of	**Z86.2**
V10.81 Bone Tumor, Hx of	**Z85.830**
V10.85 Brain Tumor, Hx of	**Z85.841**
V15.1 Cardiovascular Surgery, Hx of	**Z98.89**
V12.54 Cerebral Infarction w/o Residual Deficits (Intrauterine Stroke), Hx of	**Z86.73**
V12.42 CNS Infection, Hx of	**Z86.61**
V13.67 Congenital Malformations of Digestive System, Hx of (Corrected)	**Z87.738**
V13.64 Congenital Malformations of Eye, Ear, Face, and Neck, Hx of (Corrected)	**Z87.730** Cleft Palate/Lip **Z87.721** Ear **Z87.720** Eye **Z87.790** Face/Neck
V13.65 Congenital Malformations of Heart and Circulatory System, Hx of (Corrected)	**Z87.74**
V13.68 Congenital Malformations of Integument, Limbs, and Musculoskeletal System, Hx of (Corrected)	**Z87.76**
V13.63 Congenital Malformations of Nervous System, Hx of (Corrected)	**Z87.728**
V13.62 Congenital Malformations of Other GU System, Hx of (Corrected)	**Z87.718**
V13.66 Congenital Malformations of Respiratory System, Hx of (Corrected)	**Z87.75**
V13.69 Congenital Malformations, Other, Hx of (Corrected)	**Z87.798**
V15.42 Emotional Abuse, Hx of	**Z62.811**

ICD-9-CM		ICD-10-CM
V12.29	Endocrine Disorder, Hx of Diabetes Mellitus	Z86.39
V15.87	Extracorporeal Membrane Oxygenation, Hx of	Z92.81
V13.61	Hypospadias, Hx of (Corrected)	Z87.710
V12.29	Immune Disorder, Hx of excludes HIV and allergy	Z86.2
V87.46	Immunosuppressive Therapy, Hx of	Z92.25
V15.22	In Utero Procedure While a Fetus, Hx of	Z98.871
V13.4	Juvenile Rheumatoid Arthritis, Hx of	Z87.39
V10.61	Leukemia, Lymphoid, Hx of	Z85.6
V10.63	Leukemia, Monocytic, Hx of	Z85.6
V10.62	Leukemia, Myeloid, Hx of	Z85.6
V10.72	Lymphoma, Hodgkin, Hx of	Z85.71
V10.71	Lymphoma, Non-Hodgkin, Hx of	Z85.72
V12.29	Metabolic Disorder, Hx of	Z86.39
V11.9	Mental Disorder, Hx of	Z65.8
V87.42	Monoclonal Drug Therapy, Hx of	Z92.22
V12.04	MRSA Infection, Hx of	Z86.14
V13.03	Nephrotic Syndrome, Hx of	Z87.441
V10.88	Neuroblastoma, Hx of	Z85.858
V12.49	Neurologic Disorder, Hx of	Z86.69
V12.1	Nutritional Deficiency, Hx of	Z86.39
V87.49	Other Drug Therapy, Hx of	Z92.29
V13.7	Perinatal Problems, Hx of excludes LBW	Z87.898
V15.41	Physical Abuse, Hx of Child Physical/Sexual Abuse Rape	Z62.810
V12.61	Pneumonia (Recurrent), Hx of	Z87.01
V15.49	Psychological Trauma, Hx of	Z91.49

V Codes: Classification of Factors Influencing Health Status and Contact With Health Services *(cont)*

ICD-9-CM		ICD-10-CM
Past Medical History Affecting Health (History Of:) (Supplementary Code) *(cont)*		
V12.69	Respiratory Disease, Other, Hx of	Z86.09
V12.60	Respiratory Disease, Unspec, Hx of	Z86.09
V10.84	Retinoblastoma, Hx of	Z85.840
V87.44	Steroid Therapy, Inhaled, Hx of	Z92.240
V87.45	Steroid Therapy, Systemic, Hx of	Z92.241
V12.53	Sudden Cardiac Arrest, Hx of	Z86.74
V12.01	TB, Hx of	Z86.11
V15.82	Tobacco Use, Hx of	Z87.891
V15.52	Traumatic Brain Injury, Hx of	Z87.820
V15.83	Under-immunization Status, Hx of Delinquent Immunizations Lapsed Immunizations	Z28.3
V13.00	Urinary Disorders, Unspec, Hx of	Z87.448
V10.52	Wilms Tumor, Hx of	Z85.528

ICD-9-CM		ICD-10-CM
Family History (Supplementary Code)		
V19.6	Allergic Conditions, Family Hx of	Z84.89
V17.6	Allergic Rhinitis/Hay Fever, Family Hx of	Z83.6
V17.7	Arthritis, Family Hx of	Z82.61
V17.5	Asthma, Family Hx of	Z82.5
V18.3	Blood Disorders, Family Hx of Sickle Cell Disease	Z83.2
V16.3	Breast Cancer, Family Hx of	Z80.3
V17.3	Cardiac Risk Factor, Family Hx of	Z82.49
V16.40	Cervical/Uterine Cancer, Family Hx of	Z80.49
V18.51	Colonic Polyps, Family Hx of	Z83.71
V18.0	Diabetes Mellitus, Family Hx of	Z83.3
V18.19	Endocrine and Metabolic Diseases, Other, Family Hx of Hypercholesterolemia	Z83.49
V18.9	Genetic Disease Carrier, Family Hx of	Z84.81

ICD-9-CM		ICD-10-CM
V19.11	Glaucoma, Family Hx of	Z83.511
V19.2	Hearing Impairment, Family Hx of	Z82.2
V18.4	Intellectual Disabilities, Family Hx of	Z81.Ø
V18.69	Kidney Disease, Other, Family Hx of	Z84.1
V16.51	Kidney Neoplasm, Family Hx of	Z80.51
V18.61	Kidney, Polycystic, Family Hx of	Z82.71
V16.6	Leukemia, Family Hx of	Z80.6
V16.7	Lymphoma, Family Hx of	Z80.7
V18.11	Multiple Endocrine Neoplasia Syndrome, Family Hx of	Z83.41
V17.89	Musculoskeletal Disease, Family Hx of	Z82.69
V16.9	Neoplasm, Unspec, Family Hx of	Z80.9
V16.8	Neurofibromatosis, Family Hx of	Z80.8
V17.2	Neurologic Disorders, Family Hx of Epilepsy	Z82.Ø
V17.81	Osteoporosis, Family Hx of	Z82.62
V19.8	Other Conditions, Family Hx of Immunosuppression	Z84.89
V17.Ø	Psychiatric Problems, Family Hx of	Z81.8
V17.41	Sudden Cardiac Death, Family Hx of	Z84.41
V19.Ø	Visual Impairment, Family Hx of	Z82.1

E Codes: Classification of External Causes of Injury, Poisoning, and Other Adverse Effects

ICD-10-CM codes are not valid for use at the time of publication and should not be reported until the official implementation date set by the Centers for Medicare & Medicaid Services.

ICD-9-CM		ICD-10-CM	
Injury Mechanism/Circumstance			
E904.0	Abandoned Newborn/Child	T74.02X√+	*perpetrator Y07.-*
E886.0	Accidental Fall From Collision, Pushing, or Shoving Playing Sports	W03.XXX√	
E917.5	Accidental Hit by Object in Sports w/ Subsequent Fall	W18.01X√	
E917.0	Accidental Hit by Object or Person in Sports w/o Fall	W21.-√	Object
		W05.XXX√	Person
E845.9	Accidental Hit by Spacecraft	V95.49X√	
E906.5	Animal Bite, Unspec	W55.81X√	
E905.5	Ant Bite	T63.421√	Accidental
E007.3	Baseball	Y93.64X√+	*place of occurrence Y92.- and status Y99.-*
E007.6	Basketball	Y93.67X√+	*place of occurrence Y92.- and status Y99.-*
E960.0	Beating/Brawl/Fight	Y04.0XX√	
E905.3	Bee/Hornet/Wasp Sting	T63.441√	Accidental, Bee
		T63.451√	Accidental, Hornet
		T63.461√	Accidental, Wasp
E826.1	Bicycle Accident, Cyclist Injured	V10.0XX√	Nontraffic
		V10.4XX√	Traffic
E826.0	Bicycle Accident, Pedestrian Injured	V01.00X√	
E006.4	Bicycle Riding	Y93.55X√+	*place of occurrence Y92.- and status Y99.-*
E812.6	Bicyclist Hit by Vehicle	V13.0XX√	Nontraffic
		V13.4XX√	Traffic
E905.9	*Bite/Sting, Unspec*	T63.441√	
E004.3	Bungee Jumping	Y93.34X√+	*place of occurrence Y92.- and status Y99.-*
E007.8	Capture the Flag	Y93.6AX√+	*place of occurrence Y92.- and status Y99.-*
E906.3	Cat Bite	W55.01X√	
E918	Caught Accidentally In or Between Objects Rock and Hard Place	W23.0XX√	

ICD-9-CM		ICD-10-CM	
E005.4	Cheerleading	Y93.45X√+	*place of occurrence Y92.- and status Y99.-*
E967.4	Child Abuse by Child	Y07.50X√	
E967.2	Child Abuse by Female Partner Child's Parent/Guardian	Y07.434√	
		Y07.14X√	Adoptive Mother
		Y07.12X√	Biological Mother
		Y07.421√	Foster Mother
		Y07.433√	Stepmother
E967.6	Child Abuse by Grandparent	Y07.499√	
E967.0	Child Abuse by Male Partner Child's Parent/Guardian	Y07.432√	
		Y07.13X√	Adoptive Father
		Y07.11X√	Biological Father
		Y07.420√	Foster Father
		Y07.430√	Stepfather
E967.8	Child Abuse by Non-related Caregiver	Y07.510√	At-Home Child Care
		Y07.511√	Day Care Center
		Y07.519√	Unspec Child Care
E967.7	Child Abuse by Other Relative	Y07.499√	
E967.1	Child Abuse by Other Specified Person	Y07.59X√	
E967.5	Child Abuse by Sibling	Y07.410√	
		Y07.435√	Stepbrother
		Y07.436√	Stepsister
E011.0	Computer Keyboarding	Y93.C1X√+	*place of occurrence Y92.- and status Y99.-*
E015.2	Cooking and Baking	Y93.G3√+	*place of occurrence Y92.- and status Y99.-*
E927.4	Cumulative Trauma From Repetitive Impact	N/A	
E927.3	Cumulative Trauma From Repetitive Motion	N/A	
E007.8	Dodgeball	Y93.6AX√+	*place of occurrence Y92.- and status Y99.-*
E906.0	Dog Bite	W54.0XX√	

E Codes: Classification of External Causes of Injury, Poisoning, and Other Adverse Effects *(cont)*

ICD-9-CM		ICD-10-CM	
Injury Mechanism/Circumstance *(cont)*			
E910.4	Drowning/Submersion, Bathtub	W56.XXX√	Accidental
E910.9	Drowning/Submersion, Swimming Pool	W67.XXX√	Accidental
E925.9	*Electric Shock*	W86.0XX√	From Home Wiring and Appliances
E927.2	**Excessive Physical Exertion From Prolonged Activity**	N/A	
E888.9	*Fall*	W19.0XX√	
E880.9	Fall Down Stairs	W10.8XX√	
E884.4	Fall From Bed	W06.XXX√	
E884.5	Fall From Changing Table	W08.XXX√	
E884.0	Fall From Playground Equipment	W09.2XX√	Jungle Gym
		W09.8XX√	Other
		W09.0XX√	Slide
		W09.1XX√	Swing
E885.1	Fall From Roller Skates, Heelies, Wheelies	V00.111√	In-line Skates
		V00.121√	Non–in-line Skates (Roller Skates)
		V00.151√	Heelies (Wheelies)
E884.9	Fall Out of Tree	W14.XXX√	
E882	Fall Out of Window	W13.4XX√	
E899	*Fire*	X08.8XX√	Unspec
E923.0	Fireworks Accident	W39.XXX√	
E007.1	Football, Flag	Y93.64X√+	*place of occurrence Y92.- and status Y99.-*
E007.0	Football, Tackle	Y93.61X√+	*place of occurrence Y92.- and status Y99.-*
E008.3	Frisbee	Y93.7XX√+	*place of occurrence Y92.- and status Y99.-*
E006.2	Golf	Y93.53X√+	*place of occurrence Y92.- and status Y99.-*
E968.6	Gun Wound, Air/Pellet Gun	X95.01X√	
E985.0	Gun Wound, Handgun	X93.XXX√	
E965.2	Gun Wound, Hunting Rifle	X94.1XX√	
E985.1	Gun Wound, Shotgun	X94.0XX√	

ICD-9-CM		ICD-10-CM	
E005.2	Gymnastics	Y93.43X√+	*place of occurrence Y92.- and status Y99.-*
E928.4	Hair Tourniquet	W49.01X√	
E011.1	Handheld Interactive Electronic Device	Y93.C2X√+	*place of occurrence Y92.- and status Y99.-*
E004.4	Hang Gliding	Y93.53X √+	*place of occurrence Y92.- and status Y99.-*
E928.6	Harmful Algae and Toxins	T65.821√	Accidental
E844.9	Hit by Falling Spacecraft	V97.89X√	
E006.1	Horseback Rider Injured	Y93.52X√+	*place of occurrence Y92.- and status Y99.-*
E928.3	Human Bite, Accidental	W50.3XX√	
E968.7	Human Bite, Intentional	Y04.1XX√	
E003.1	Ice Hockey	Y93.22X√+	*place of occurrence Y92.- and status Y99.-*
E960.0	Injured by Audience for Failing to Silence or Using Cell Phone During an Event	Y04.0XX	
E906.9	Injury by Animal	W64.XXX√	
E906.4	Insect Bite (Nonvenomous)	W57.XXX√	
E905.6	Jellyfish Sting	T63.621√	Accidental
E920.3	Knife Wound, Accidental	W26.0XX√	
E966	Knife Wound, Intentional	X78.1XX√	
E012.0	Knitting and Crocheting	Y93.D1X√+	*place of occurrence Y92.- and status Y99.-*
E007.4	Lacrosse and Field Hockey	Y93.65√+	*place of occurrence Y92.- and status Y99.-*
E013.1	Laundry	Y93.E2X√+	*place of occurrence Y92.- and status Y99.-*
E920.0	Lawn Mower Accident	W28.XXX√	
E019.1	Milking an Animal	Y93.K2√+	*place of occurrence Y92.- and status Y99.-*
E819.9	*Motor Vehicle Accident*	V43.-√	
E812.0	Motor Vehicle Collision, Driver Injured	V43.-√	
E812.2	Motor Vehicle Collision, Motorcyclist Injured	V23.-√	

E Codes: Classification of External Causes of Injury, Poisoning, and Other Adverse Effects *(cont)*

ICD-9-CM		ICD-10-CM	
Injury Mechanism/Circumstance *(cont)*			
E812.1	Motor Vehicle Collision, Passenger Injured	**V43.-√**	
E812.3	Motor Vehicle Collision, Passenger on Motorcycle Injured	**V29.59X√**	
E920.5	Needlestick	**W46.0XX√**	
E821.9	*Off-road Vehicle Accident*	**V86.99X√**	
E821.0	Off-road Vehicle Accident, Driver Injured ATV Driver	**V86.09X√**	
E821.2	Off-road Vehicle Accident, Motorcyclist Injured	**V88.8XX√**	
E821.0	Off-road Vehicle Accident, Passenger Injured ATV Passenger	**V86.19X√**	
E821.3	Off-road Vehicle Accident, Passenger on Motorcycle Injured	**V88.8XX√**	
E927.0	Overexertion From Sudden Strenuous Movement	**N/A**	
E922.5	Paintball Gun	**X95.02X√**	
E814.7	Pedestrian Hit by Vehicle	**V03.10X√**	
E018.0	Piano Playing	**Y93.J1X√+**	*place of occurrence Y92.- and status Y99.-*
E010.3	Pilates	**Y93.B4√X+**	*place of occurrence Y92.- and status Y99.-*
E960.1	Rape	**Y04.8XX√**	
E029.0	Refereeing a Sports Activity	**Y93.81X√+**	*place of occurrence Y92.- and status Y99.-*
E017.0	Roller Coaster Riding	**Y93.I1X√+**	*place of occurrence Y92.- and status Y99.-*
E006.0	Roller-skating (In-line) and Skateboarding	**Y93.51X√+**	*place of occurrence Y92.- and status Y99.-*
E029.2	Roughhousing and Horseplay	**Y93.83X√+**	*place of occurrence Y92.- and status Y99.-*
E007.2	Rugby	**Y93.62X√+**	*place of occurrence Y92.- and status Y99.-*
E001.1	Running	**Y93.02X√+**	*place of occurrence Y92.- and status Y99.-*

ICD-9-CM		ICD-10-CM	
E890.2	Smoke Inhalation, House Fire	X02.1XX√	Controlled
		X00.1XX√	Uncontrolled
E905.0	Snakebite	T63.001√	Snake, Unspec, Accidental
E820.9	*Snowmobile Accident*	Y93.29X√+	*place of occurrence Y92.- and status Y99.-*
E007.5	Soccer	Y93.66X√+	*place of occurrence Y92.- and status Y99.-*
E029.1	Spectator at Event	Y93.82X√+	*place of occurrence Y92.- and status Y99.-*
E905.1	Spider (Venomous) Bite	T63.301√	Spider, Unspec, Accidental
E917.0	Sports Related	W21.89X√	
E920.8	Stepped on Nail	W45.8XX√	
E916	Struck (by Object) Accidentally	W20.8XX√	
E002.7	Surfing, Windsurfing, and Boogie Boarding	Y93.18X√+	*place of occurrence Y92.- and status Y99.-*
E002.0	Swimming	Y93.11	
E005.3	Trampoline	Y93.44X√+	*place of occurrence Y92.- and status Y99.-*
E926.2	Visible and Ultraviolet Light	W89.8XX√	
E007.7	Volleyball	Y93.68X√+	*place of occurrence Y92.- and status Y99.-*
E002.5	Water Activities	Y93.19X√+	*place of occurrence Y92.- and status Y99.-*
	Rowing, Canoeing, Kayaking, Rafting, Tubing	Y93.16X√+	*place of occurrence Y92.- and status Y99.-*
E924.0	Water Burn/Scald, Boiling/Steam	X13.0XX√	Inhalation Steam
		X13.1XX√	Other
E924.2	Water Burn/Scald, Tap	X11.0XX√	Bath or Tub
		X11.8XX√	Other Hot Tap Water
		X11.1XX√	Running Hot Water (Including Bathtub)
E838.9	*Watercraft Accident*	V94.89X√	
E002.6	Waterskiing and Wakeboarding	Y93.17X√+	*place of occurrence Y92.- and status Y99.-*

E Codes: Classification of External Causes of Injury, Poisoning, and Other Adverse Effects *(cont)*

ICD-9-CM		ICD-10-CM	
Injury Mechanism/Circumstance *(cont)*			
E008.1	Wrestling	Y93.72X√+	*place of occurrence Y92.- and status Y99.-*
E005.1	Yoga	Y93.42X√+	*place of occurrence Y92.- and status Y99.-*

Adverse Effects (Including Allergic Reaction), Not Due to an Accidental Ingestion or Intentional Misuse			
E935.4	Acetaminophen	T39.1X5√	
E945.7	Albuterol	T48.6X5√	
E930.8	Antibiotics, Other	T36.8X5√	
E933.0	Antihistamines/Antiemetics	T45.0X5√	
E934.7	Blood Products	T80.319√	Unspec ABO Incompatibility
E930.5	Cephalosporins	T36.1X5√	
E937.1	Chloral Hydrate	T42.6X5√	
E935.2	Codeine/Morphine/Opiates	T40.2X5√	
E945.6	Cold Remedies	T48.5X5√	
E945.4	Dextromethorphan	T48.3X5√	
E941.2	Epinephrine	T44.5X5√	
E930.3	Erythromycin/Macrolides	T36.3X5√	
E935.6	Ibuprofen/Naproxen	T39.395√	
E939.0	Imipramine	T43.025√	
E932.3	Insulin/Antidiabetic Agents	T38.3X5√	
E932.8	Iodides	T38.2X5√	
E934.0	Iron Compounds	T45.4X5√	
E933.0	Metoclopramide	T47.8X5√	
E930.0	Penicillins	T36.0X5√	
E948.6	Pertussis Vaccine	T50.A15√	
E939.1	Phenothiazines	T43.595√	
E936.1	Phenytoin	T42.0X5√	
E930.6	Rifampin	T36.6X5√	
E935.3	Salicylates	T39.094√	
E931.0	Sulfonamide	T37.0X5√	
E948.8	Vaccine, Bacterial, Other	T50.A95√	
E949.6	Vaccine, Viral/Rickettsial	T50.B95√	